MW01064763

Institute on Science for Global Policy (ISGP)

Emerging and Persistent Infectious Diseases:
Focus on the Societal and Economic Context

Conference convened by the ISGP at George Mason University

Fairfax, Virginia, U.S.

July 8-11, 2012

An ongoing series of dialogues and critical debates
examining the role of science and technology
in advancing effective domestic and international policy decisions

Institute on Science for Global Policy (ISGP)

Tucson, AZ Office
845 N. Park Ave., 5th Floor
PO Box 210158-B
Tucson, AZ 85721

Washington, DC Office
818 Connecticut Ave. NW
Suite 800
Washington, DC 20006

www.scienceforglobalpolicy.org

ISBN: 978-0-9830882-3-3

Table of contents

iv

Introduction

Dr. George H. Atkinson
Founder and Executive Director, Institute on Science for Global Policy
and
Professor Emeritus, Department of Chemistry and Biochemistry
and College of Optical Sciences,
University of Arizona

Preface

The contents of this book were taken from material presented at an international conference convened by the Institute on Science for Global Policy (ISGP) on July 8-11, 2012 at George Mason University in Fairfax, Virginia. This ISGP conference specifically addressed the social, economic, and ethical considerations of the largely scientific and technological recommendations that emerged from four earlier ISGP conferences focused on Emerging and Persistent Infectious Diseases (EPID). Aspects of Food Safety and Security (FSS) and Synthetic Biology (SB) related to infectious diseases were also addressed.

It is important to clarify the relationship between the initial four ISGP conferences focused on EPID, FSS, and SB and the ISGP conference convened at George Mason University. The recommendations (i.e., the specific areas of consensus and actionable next steps are published in the respective ISGP books for each conference) emerging from the initial four conferences offered primarily scientific and technological options to be considered by those responsible for formulating and implementing policies, both domestic and international. Since the effectiveness of such policy decisions depends fundamentally on the degree to which they are accepted and endorsed throughout a wide range of societies and cultures, it is essential to evaluate these recommendations with respect to their foreseeable societal, economic, and ethical impact. The public support required to effectively implement these largely scientific and technological recommendations depends directly on the societal, economic, and ethical consequences that can influence public acceptance.

The ISGP invited eight highly distinguished subject-matter experts working on social, behavioral, economic, and ethical topics to prepare the policy position papers debated at this ISGP conference. To aid these authors, the ISGP prepared a new document that condensed all the previous recommendations into four areas of consensus and their related actionable next steps. This document, presented at the end of this introduction, was shared with each of the presenters as a guideline for their individual policy position papers.

The material in this book includes policy position papers prepared by eight internationally distinguished socio-behavioral scientists, economists, and ethicists together with the not-for-attribution summaries prepared by the ISGP staff of the discussions, debates, and caucuses that comprised the ISGP conference. While the material presented here is comprehensive and stands by itself, its policy significance is best appreciated if viewed within the context of how domestic and international science policies have been, and often currently are being, formulated and implemented.

Current realities

As the second decade of the 21st century opens, most societies are facing difficult decisions concerning how to appropriately use, or reject, the dramatic new opportunities offered by modern scientific advances and the technologies that emanate from them. Advanced scientific research programs, as well as commercially viable technologies, are now developed globally. As a consequence, many societal issues related to science and technology (S&T) necessarily involve both domestic and international policy decisions. The daunting challenges to simultaneously recognize immediate technological opportunities, while identifying those emerging and "at-the-horizon" S&T achievements that foreshadow transformational advantages and risks within specific societies, are now fundamental governmental responsibilities. These responsibilities are especially complex since policy makers must consider the demands of different segments of society often having conflicting goals. For example, decisions must balance critical commercial interests that promote economic prosperity with the cultural sensitivities that often determine if, and how, S&T can be successfully integrated into any society.

Many of our most significant geopolitical policy and security issues are directly connected with the remarkably rapid and profound S&T accomplishments of our time. Consequently, it is increasingly important that the S&T and policy communities communicate effectively. With a seemingly unlimited number of urgent S&T challenges, both wealthy and less-wealthy societies need the most accomplished members of these communities to focus on effective, real-world solutions relevant to their specific circumstances. Some of the most prominent challenges involve (i) infectious diseases and pandemics, (ii) environmentally compatible energy sources, (iii) the consequences of climate change, (iv) food safety, security, and defense, (v) the cultural impact of stem cell applications, (vi) nanotechnology and human health, (vii) cyber security for advanced telecommunication, (viii) the security implications of quantum computing, and (ix) the cultural radicalization of societies.

Recent history suggests that most societies would benefit from improving the effectiveness of how scientifically credible information is used to formulate and implement governmental and private sector policies, both domestic and international. Specifically, there is a critical need to have the relevant S&T information concisely presented to policy communities in an environment that promotes candid questions and debates led by those non-experts directly engaged in policy decisions. Such discussions, sequestered away from publicity, can help to clarify the advantages and potential risks of realistic S&T options directly relevant to the challenges being faced. Eventually, this same degree of understanding, confidence, and acknowledgment of risk must be communicated to the public to obtain the broad societal support needed to effectively implement any decision.

The ISGP mission

The Institute on Science for Global Policy (ISGP) has pioneered the development of a new type of international forum based on a series of invitation-only conferences. These ISGP conferences are designed to provide articulate, distinguished scientists and technologists opportunities to concisely present their views of the credible S&T options available for addressing major geopolitical and security issues. Over a two-year-plus period, these ISGP conferences are convened on different aspects (e.g., surveillance, prevention, or mitigation) of a broad, overarching topic (e.g., EPID and related aspects of FSS and SB). The format used emphasizes written and oral policy-oriented S&T presentations and extensive debates led by an international cross section of the policy community.

The current realities, relevant S&T-based options (including risks), and policy issues are debated among a few scientists selected by the ISGP and an international group of government, private sector, and societal leaders selected following consultations with the participating governments and organizations. ISGP conferences reflect global perspectives and seek to provide government and community leaders with the clear, accurate understanding of the real-world challenges and potential solutions critical to determining sound public policies.

ISGP programs rely on the validity of two overarching principles:

1. Scientifically credible understanding must be closely linked to the realistic policy decisions made by governmental and societal leaders in addressing

both the urgent and long-term challenges facing 21st century societies. Effective decisions rely on strong domestic and global public endorsements that motivate active support throughout societies.

2. Communication among scientific and policy communities requires significant improvement, especially concerning decisions on whether to use or reject the often transformational scientific and technological opportunities continually emerging from the global research communities. Effective decisions are facilitated in venues where the advantages and risks of credible options are candidly presented and critically debated among internationally distinguished subject-matter experts, policy makers, and private sector and community stakeholders.

Historical perspective

The dramatic and rapid expansion of academic and private sector scientific research transformed many societies of the 20th century and is a major factor in the emergence of the more-affluent countries that currently dominate the global economic and security landscape. The positive influence of these S&T achievements has been extremely impressive and in many ways the hallmark of the 20th century. However, there have also been numerous negative consequences, some immediately apparent and others appearing only recently. From both perspectives, it would be difficult to argue that S&T has not been the prime factor defining the societies we know today. Indeed, the 20th century can be viewed through the prism of how societies decided to use the available scientific understanding and technological expertise to structure themselves. Such decisions helped shape the respective economic models, cultural priorities, and security commitments in these societies.

It remains to be seen how the prosperity and security of 21st century societies will be shaped by the decisions made by our current leaders, especially with respect to how these decisions reflect sound S&T understanding.

Given the critical importance of properly incorporating scientifically credible information into major societal decisions, it is surprising that the process by which this is achieved by the public and its political leadership has been uneven and, occasionally, haphazard. In the worst cases, decisions have been based on unrecognized misunderstanding, overhyped optimism, and/or limited respect for potentially negative consequences. Retrospectively, while some of these outcomes may be attributed to politically motivated priorities, the inability of S&T experts to accurately communicate the advantages and potential risks of a given option must also be acknowledged as equally important.

The new conference format pioneered by the ISGP in its programs seeks to facilitate candid communication between scientific and policy communities in ways that complement and support the efforts of others.

It is important to recognize that policy makers routinely seek a degree of certainty in evaluating S&T-based options that is inconsistent with reality, while S&T experts often overvalue the potentially positive aspects of their proposals. Finite uncertainty is always part of advanced scientific thinking and all possible positive outcomes in S&T proposals are rarely realized. Both points need to be reflected in policy decisions. Eventually, the public needs to be given a frank, accurate assessment of the potential advantages and foreseeable disadvantages associated with these decisions. Such disclosures are essential to obtain the broad public support required to effectively implement any major decision.

ISGP conference structure

At each ISGP conference, eight internationally recognized, subject-matter experts are invited to prepare concise (three pages) policy position papers. For the July 8-11, 2012, ISGP conference at George Mason University, these papers described the authors' views on current realities, scientifically credible opportunities and associated risks, and policy issues within the socio-economic context of earlier recommendations made at ISGP conferences on EPID, FSS, and SB.

These eight authors were chosen to represent a broad cross section of viewpoints and an international perspective. Several weeks before the conference convened, these policy position papers were distributed to representatives from governments, societal and private sector organizations, and international organizations engaged with the ISGP (the United States, Italy, the United Kingdom, Japan, Canada, Switzerland, Germany, the Food and Agricultural Organization of the United Nations, and the European Commission). Individuals from several private sector and philanthropic organizations also were invited to participate and, therefore, received the papers.

The conference agenda was comprised of eight 90-minute sessions, each of which was devoted to a debate of a given policy position paper. To encourage frank discussions and critical debates, all ISGP conferences are conducted under the Chatham House Rule (i.e., all the information can be used freely, but there can be no attribution of any remark to any participant outside the conference). In each session, the author was given 5 minutes to summarize his or her views while the remaining 85 minutes were opened to all participants, including other authors, for questions, comments, and debate. The focus was on obtaining clarity of understanding among the nonspecialists and identifying areas of consensus and actionable policy decisions supported by scientifically credible information. With active participation from North America, Europe, and Asia, these candid debates are designed to reflect international perspectives on real-world problems.

The ISGP staff attended the debates of all eight policy position papers. The "not-for-attribution" summaries of each debate, prepared from their collective notes, are presented here immediately following each policy position paper. These summaries represent the ISGP's best effort to accurately capture the comments and questions made by the participants, including the other authors, as well as those responses made by the author of the paper. The views expressed in these summaries do not necessarily represent the views of a specific author, as evidenced by his or her respective policy position paper. Rather, the summaries are, and should be read as, an overview of the areas of agreement and disagreement that emerged from all those participating in the debates.

Separate caucuses were held after the eight debates for small groups of the participants. A separate caucus for the scientific presenters also was held. These caucuses focused on identifying areas of consensus and actionable next steps for consideration within governments and civil societies in general. Subsequently, a plenary caucus was convened for all participants. While the debates focused on specific issues and recommendations raised in each policy position paper, the caucuses focused on overarching views and conclusions that could have policy relevance both domestically and internationally.

A summary of the overall areas of consensus and actionable next steps emerging from these caucuses is presented here immediately following this introduction under the title of **Conference conclusions.**

Concluding remarks

ISGP conferences are designed to provide new and unusual (perhaps unique) environments that facilitate and encourage candid debate of the credible S&T options vital to successfully address many of the most significant challenges facing 21st century societies. ISGP debates test the views of subject-matter experts through critical questions and comments from an international group of decision makers committed to finding effective, real-world solutions. Obviously, ISGP conferences build on the authoritative reports and expertise expressed by many domestic and international organizations already actively devoted to this task. The ISGP has no preconceived opinions nor do members of the ISGP staff express any independent views on these topics. Rather, ISGP programs focus on fostering environments that can significantly improve the communication of ideas and recommendations, many of which are in reports developed by other organizations and institutes, to the policy communities responsible for serving their constituents.

ISGP conferences begin with concise descriptions of scientifically credible options provided by those experienced in the S&T subject, but rely heavily on the willingness of nonspecialists in government, academe, foundations, and the private sector to critically debate these S&T concepts and proposals. Overall, ISGP conferences seek to provide a new type of venue in which S&T expertise not only informs the nonspecialists, but also in which the debates and caucuses identify realistic policy options for serious consideration by governments and societal leaders. These new ISGP programs can help ensure that S&T understanding is integrated into those real-world policy decisions needed to foster safer and more prosperous 21st century societies.

Condensed areas of consensus and actionable next steps from the four previous ISGP conferences

1. Emerging and Persistent Infectious Diseases (EPID):

Area of consensus

The potential for infectious diseases, known and emerging, to reach pandemic levels has been credibly characterized as "not if, but when." The negative consequences of a pandemic for human health and mortality, the functioning of modern economic systems, and even geopolitical stability worldwide would constitute a major threat to the security and prosperity of not only the United States, but essentially all societies. Infectious diseases, however, remain largely under-recognized as a significant, urgent priority within many policy communities. Therefore, the scale of resources and governmental attention required to establish the global commitment necessary to even ameliorate the anticipated risks have yet to be made. To effectively address the ongoing impact of infectious diseases as it pertains to pandemics, policies must accurately reflect (i) the continuously expanding, scientifically credible understanding of how diseases originate and transmit among animals and humans and (ii) international perspectives on how preventive and clinical approaches are accepted or rejected based on diverse cultures and economic systems. Specific resources in support of more proactive policies are needed to foster globally integrated programs for laboratory research, real-world surveillance, and the infrastructure in support of the rapid development of drugs and vaccines. Special attention must be given to the well-recognized importance of the surveillance and treatment of the animal diseases that are recognized as major sources of human diseases.

Actionable next steps

1.1 Information sharing:

Surveillance data, epidemiological findings, microbiological materials (e.g., samples), and recommendations pertaining to disease prevention and mitigation must be shared rapidly and in a transparent manner, within countries, between countries, and across professional disciplines.

- To ensure that actionable decisions are implemented by governments and societal organizations, disease surveillance data need to be standardized for content and format, and rapidly shared among networks of health professionals at local, regional, national, and international levels.

- Coordinated systems for sharing best practices and recommendations concerning the prevention and mitigation of infectious diseases are required to dramatically reduce duplicated efforts in field programs, optimize the allocation of limited human and financial resources, and maximize the societal impact of subsequent analyses and modeling.

- Evolving technologies and communication tools (e.g., social networking, "crowd-sourcing," contact tracing, and mining of Twitter feeds) must be more effectively used for (i) the surveillance of disease dynamics and population behavior and (ii) the public dissemination of information for disease prevention and mitigation.

1.2 One Health:

The effectiveness of infectious disease surveillance, prevention, and mitigation strategies depends on a greater commitment to the One Health approach involving collaborations among the communities addressing human, animal, and wildlife health.

- An independent organization with global coordinating responsibilities and unified leadership, supported at the highest levels of governmental, private sector, and societal leadership, is needed to establish One Health efforts at the local, national, regional, and international levels.

- To strengthen the effectiveness of One Health initiatives, institutional and professional priorities and strategies, budgetary requests and expenditures, terminologies, methodologies, and data collection efforts must be coordinated among agencies responsible for human, animal, and wildlife health.

- Internationally endorsed standards, that take into account the influence of environmental conditions, social and cultural perspectives, ecological characteristics, and economic factors on the appearance and transmission of infectious diseases must be developed for the education of One Health practitioners.

- It is critical to establish public-private partnerships committed to increasing the resources available for One Health.

2. Food safety and security (FSS):

Area of consensus

Providing nutritious food, an essential commodity for all humans, has become one of the highest priorities for policy makers worldwide. The unprecedented increase in the human population (9 billion by 2040), together with changing dietary habits, demands a new international supply system that substantially increases the amount of healthy food, feed, and fiber currently produced (i.e., double by 2040). Food safety and security (i.e., an adequate supply of nutritious food free from accidental and/or intentional contamination), has become an increasingly critical governmental responsibility in promoting domestic, and potentially global, stability.

Immediate and major improvements are required in (i) efforts to understand the global food supply chain, (ii) speed and accuracy with which food pathogens and their vehicles are identified, (iii) corrective policies and interventions used when foodborne pathogens appear in the food supply chain, especially the sharing of data across agencies and borders, and (iv) molecular diagnostics, production technologies, and risk assessments tools available to support surveillance for and testing of foodborne diseases. Such improvements, based on governmental recognition of the significance of food issues in the promotion of national security and economic prosperity, require renewed commitments of resources and support for policies that ensure international regulation.

Actionable next steps

Preventing and mitigating foodborne diseases, and minimizing the associated economic impact, depend on significantly improving surveillance of foodborne pathogens through the accurate and rapid identification of the sources of contamination.

- A comprehensive and global source attribution system is needed that correctly identifies and characterizes microbes in the food chain, especially those that are pathogenic to humans. The effectiveness of such a system critically depends on incorporating emerging technology (e.g., DNA sequencing, radio frequency identification tags) and capacity building in resource-poor regions of the world (i.e., providing state-of-the-art training and equipment).

- To effectively ensure the safety of the world's food supply, the food industry and governments must jointly develop substantially more harmonized standards, regulations, and guidelines for food safety, and globally implement comprehensive protocols to effectively prevent and mitigate foodborne diseases.

- Government and industry strategies need to shift from hazard-based to risk-based approaches if resources for the prevention and mitigation of foodborne diseases are to be maximized.

3. Synthetic Biology (SB):

Area of consensus

Synthetic biology, the most recent manifestation of the often-transformational advances in biotechnology (e.g., nanomedicine, stem cell applications, and genetically modified organisms) is rapidly redefining many social and commercial aspects of 21st century societies. Synthetic biology has the realistic potential of altering national security postures in the United States and worldwide, both from a physical and economic perspective. The acceptance or rejection of the dramatic benefits to human health foreseen by researchers to be within reach must be viewed as part of governmental and societal responsibilities to appropriately regulate for public use. The use of synthetic biology can be reasonably anticipated to significantly influence economic prosperity worldwide and perhaps cause major restructurings throughout global societies.

Actionable next step

Managing the intended and unintended consequences of synthetic biology applications requires balanced governmental scrutiny to preserve opportunities for constructive innovation while minimizing the potential for negative impact on national security, economic prosperity, and public health.

- The widely recognized benefits and potential harm, deliberate or accidental, associated with synthetic biology require government and the private sector to jointly create regulatory and safety frameworks that nurture innovation, improve human health, protect public safety, maintain national security, and promote economic prosperity. The training of all professional and amateur practitioners of synthetic biology, supervised and unsupervised, must include certified guidelines on biosafety, biosecurity, and codes of ethical conduct and must be based on coherent definitions of synthetic biology.

4. Communication:

Area of consensus

The communication to the lay public of accurate, consistent, and timely information from scientists, public officials, and authoritative policy makers remains the most pervasive and underdeveloped element critical to effectively implementing any policies related to scientifically credible information. A strategically coordinated plan for formulating and transmitting accurate information from publicly trusted sources is currently absent in most communities worldwide. Fundamental to the process is the rapid sharing of surveillance, diagnostic, and analysis data among myriad agencies, departments, and municipalities now empowered to communicate publicly. Presenting confusing and contradictory messages undermines essentially all preparatory efforts and minimizes the potential that even effective policies are properly implemented.

Actionable next step

Improved communication requires proactive consensus building to develop messages, and significantly enhanced training and evaluation to strengthen the communication skills of the science, technology, and policy communities.

- Messages and recommendations concerning disease prevention and mitigation can be effectively disseminated only if the communication skills of those responsible for conveying them to the public are significantly improved. The complexity and volume of the disease information, and the rapidity with which it becomes available, demand clear, evidence-based messages to the public be proactively coordinated among government, industry, and mass media.

Conference conclusions

1. Emerging and Persistent Infectious Diseases

Area of consensus

Emerging and persistent infectious diseases remain largely under-recognized within many policy communities as an urgent priority demanding immediate attention and the allocation of significant resources. To effectively address the ongoing impact of infectious diseases, including as it pertains to pandemics, policies need to: (i) accurately reflect the continuously expanding, scientifically credible understanding of how diseases originate and transmit among animals and humans, (ii) build on international perspectives concerning the importance of differences in cultures and economic systems, (iii) promote multidisciplinary collaborations, (iv) invest in global capacity building for research, surveillance, and infrastructure to aid in the rapid development and deployment of diagnostics, vaccines, and drugs, and (v) focus on the critical contributions animal and environmental factors make in the acquisition and spread of infectious diseases in humans.

Actionable next steps

1.1 Information sharing:

- Rapidly share actionable disease surveillance data in usable formats among response networks at local, regional, national, and international levels. Methods for improving disease surveillance capacities are prioritized in international agreements (e.g., the International Health Regulations and the Performance of Veterinary Services). Optimize the sharing of surveillance data, best practices, and analysis methods to eliminate duplicative effort and optimize the allocation of limited human and financial resources.

- Expand the use of both traditional and rapidly evolving modern communication technologies (e.g., social networking, crowd-sourcing, contact tracing, and mining electronic communication feeds) to improve the surveillance of disease dynamics and population behavior as well as the public dissemination of credible information from trusted sources.

1.2 One Health:

- Strengthen leadership commitments at all levels to those interdisciplinary, multi-stakeholder, and international efforts that integrate human, animal, and ecological health issues into the prevention, mitigation, and control of infectious diseases **in humans**.

- Expand the global coordination of and support for locally prioritized solutions based on a credible understanding of how human, animal, and ecological factors influence **human health**.

- Align interdisciplinary collaborations that manage data, allocate resources, and commit funding among public and private entities responsible for human, animal, wildlife, and ecological health.

- Share best practices, internationally across disciplines, for reducing the appearance and transmission of infectious diseases. These best practices must reflect the influence of environmental conditions, social and cultural perspectives, ecological characteristics, and economic factors.

2. Food Safety and Security (FSS):

Area of consensus

Food safety and security (i.e., an adequate supply of nutritious food free from accidental and/or intentional contamination) has become an increasingly critical governmental responsibility in promoting societal stability, both domestically and internationally. Immediate and major improvements are required to (i) understand the global food supply chain, (ii) increase the speed and accuracy with which food pathogens and their vectors are identified, (iii) formulate and implement policies and interventions that prevent and mitigate the impact of foodborne pathogens appearing in the food supply chain (especially concerning the sharing of data across agencies and borders), and (iv) expand and optimize the technological tools and methods available for diagnostics, production, safety interventions, and risk assessments associated with foodborne diseases. Renewed commitments of resources and support for policies that ensure international oversight and regulation are also required.

Actionable next steps

- The food industry and government urgently need to jointly implement comprehensive protocols to enhance the safety of the world's food supply by harmonizing domestic and international standards, regulations, and guidelines associated with foodborne diseases.

- Shift government and food industry strategies from hazard-based to risk-based approaches.

- Improve traceability methods based on emerging technologies to identify the source(s) of foodborne diseases in concert with strengthening the capacity in less-affluent regions to accurately characterize microbes (i.e., pathogens) in the food chain.

3. Synthetic Biology (SB):

Area of consensus

Synthetic biology has the potential to rapidly redefine many social and commercial aspects of 21st century societies by addressing significant societal challenges including food production, clean water, biofuels, and transformative treatments for human diseases. Synthetic biology can also be envisioned to be the source of harmful outcomes including organisms designed for nefarious purposes, the accidental or intentional release of synthetic pathogens, and/or the creation of organisms with unforeseen consequences. The development of synthetic biology can be reasonably anticipated to significantly alter economic prosperity worldwide, restructure global societies, and impact security postures globally.

Actionable next steps

- Coordinate the regulatory and safety frameworks formulated by governments and the private sector intended to improve human health and food productivity, protect public safety and national security, and promote innovation and economic prosperity.

- Develop educational programs for both professional and amateur practitioners of synthetic biology using certified guidelines for biosafety, biosecurity, and codes of ethical conduct reflective of best practices and legal responsibilities.

4. Communication:

Area of consensus

The prevention, mitigation, and control of the negative consequences of infectious disease outbreaks depends critically on the dissemination of accurate, timely, and credible information to the public from those responsible for messaging prior to, during, and following an event. It would be difficult to overemphasize the importance of significantly improving the skills of those involved in such communications not only with the public, but also among scientists, first responders, public officials, and policy makers.

Actionable next steps

- Develop coordinated mechanisms to provide scientifically credible, consistent, and timely messages to the public that acknowledge uncertainty where appropriate and contain the information needed by the lay person for the public to make informed decisions.

- Identify and train trusted individuals (e.g., scientists, officials, and community leaders) who can communicate infectious disease messages tailored to public perceptions of risk and differences in cultural and political viewpoints.

- Evaluate the effectiveness of messages prior to dissemination using proven empirical methods (e.g., scenario simulations and focus groups).

ISGP conference program

Sunday, June 8

12:00 – 17:00	**Arrival and Registration: The Mason Inn, George Mason University**
16:00 – 16:30	**Conference Meeting: Caucus Group Leaders and Co-Leaders**
16:30 – 17:30	**Caucus Meeting: All presenters and participants**
17:30 – 18:45	*Reception*
18:45-19:00	**Welcome Remarks**

Dr. George Atkinson, Institute on Science for Global Policy (ISGP) Founder and Executive Director

And

Dr. Roger Stough, Vice President for Research and Economic Development, George Mason University

19:00 – 20:30	*Dinner*
20:30 – 21:00	**Conference Overview**

Dr. George Atkinson, ISGP Founder and Executive Director

21:00 – 22:00	**Conference Meeting: Science Presenters**

Monday, June 9

08:00 – 08:45	*Breakfast*

Presentations and Debates: Session 1

09:00 – 10:30	**Dr. Jakob Zinsstag, Epidemiology & Public Health, Human & Animal Health, Swiss Tropical Institut, Switzerland**

One Health+: Integrated Control and Elimination of Zoonoses

10:30 – 11:00	*Break*
11:00 – 12:30	**Dr. Richard Williams, Mercatus Center, George Mason University, United States**

Solving Food Safety Problems Without Antiquated Regulation and Inspection

12:30 – 14:00	*Lunch*

Presentations and Debates: Session 2

14:00 – 15:30   **Dr. Vanessa Hayes, J. Craig Venter Institute, United States and South Africa**
Translating Technical Advances in Genomics to the Developing World: Addressing Cultural Needs as Part of Policy-Making

15:30 – 16:00   *Break*

16:00 – 17:30   **Prof. Paul Slovic, University of Oregon, United States**
Communication Challenges in Managing Social and Economic Impacts of Emerging and Infectious Diseases

19:00 – 20:00   *Dinner*

20:00 – 20:45   **Evening Remarks**
Dr. John P. Holdren, Assistant to the President for Science and Technology, Director of the White House Office of Science and Technology Policy, and Co-Chair of the President's Council of Advisors on Science and Technology (PCAST)

Tuesday, June 10

08:00 – 08:45   *Breakfast*

Presentations and Debates: Session 3

09:00 – 10:30   **Prof. Arthur Caplan, Department of Medical Ethics and Health Policy, University of Pennsylvania, United States**
Synthetic Biology: Ethical and Social Challenges

10:30 – 11:00   *Break*

11:00 – 12:30   **Dr. Peter Daszak, EcoHealth Alliance, United States and United Kingdom**
How Can We Predict, Prevent and Pay for the Next Pandemic?

12:30 – 14:00   *Lunch*

Presentations and Debates: Session 4

14:00 – 15:30   **Dr. Laura Kahn, Program on Science and Global Security at the Woodrow Wilson School of Public and International Affairs, Princeton University and One Health Initiative, United States**
The Challenges of Implementing One Health

15:30 – 16:00   *Break*

16:00 – 17:30   **Prof. Gay Miller, College of Veterinary Medicine, University of Illinois at Urbana/Champaign, United States**
Will a Comprehensive Global Source Attribution System Provide for Cost-Effective Food Safety?

Caucuses

17:30 – 22:00   **Focused group sessions**

Wednesday, June 11

08:00 – 08:45   *Breakfast*

09:00 – 12:10   **Plenary Caucus Session**
Dr. George Atkinson, *moderator*

12:10 – 12:30   **Closing Remarks, discussion of ISGP conferences 2012–2013**
Dr. George Atkinson

12:30 – 13:30   *Lunch*

13:30   *Adjournment*

One Health+: Integrated Control and Elimination of Zoonoses**

Jakob Zinsstag, D.V.M., Ph.D., Diplomate ECVPH
Deputy Head of Department Epidemiology and Public Health
Swiss Tropical and Public Health Institute and University of Basel,
Basel, Switzerland

Summary

Emerging diseases generate media and public interest in industrialized countries, yet this interest does not accurately reflect the type of infectious diseases where attention is globally most needed. It can be argued that in less-affluent nations and countries in transition, the burden of re-emerging and endemic zoonoses outweighs the burden and associated costs of emerging zoonoses. Less-affluent nations and countries in transition often have inadequate surveillance-response systems. Factors that influence the emergence and persistence of zoonoses are more fully understood at the molecular level, but there is much to be learned about the determinants of transmission at the population level in specific settings. There is currently a lack of understanding regarding intervention effectiveness across all biological, environmental, social, and psychological determinants. "One Health" has no well-defined theoretical framework. In particular, it lacks a socioeconomic perspective and is poorly implemented at the international level. My colleagues and I contend that recognition of inextricable linkages among humans, livestock, companion animals, and wildlife is a necessary requirement for One Health, but it is not sufficient. The success of One Health is dependent on the demonstration of an added value of health and well-being of humans and animals and/or financial savings from closer cooperation of human and animal health initiatives. We propose a concept built on the theory of effectiveness of interventions, combining scientific disciplines that usually work separately, and extending the theory to the animal-human interface at the population level. Understanding the determinants of the effectiveness of surveillance and interventions at different scales, ranging from the household to the government level, can then provide convincing evidence for policy and practice.

Current realities

More than 60% of all human infectious disease and 75% of all newly emerging diseases are of animal origin and are referred to as zoonoses. Disease transmission is driven, among other factors, by demographic and behavioral changes. Domestic animal populations grow in parallel to the human population, a phenomenon called the "livestock revolution," which improves economic livelihoods for hundreds of millions of farmers, but also increases susceptible host populations for transmission of zoonoses due to poor biosecurity (e.g. backyard farming). Among many other ways, zoonoses can be grouped according to the level of public consciousness elicited. In more-affluent countries, the public's attention is attracted to emerging diseases, primarily zoonoses, such as bovine spongiform encephalitis (BSE), severe acute respiratory syndrome (SARS), highly pathogenic avian influenza (HPAI), and animal-source foodborne pathogens. Much less public attention is directed toward re-emerging zoonoses, such as brucellosis and echinococcosis, which are linked to factors including the breakdown of public health systems after the socialist period ended in former countries of the Soviet Union. Also in this group are endemic zoonoses with wildlife reservoirs, such as rabies in North America and bovine tuberculosis in the United Kingdom. A small fraction of public consideration is given to endemic zoonoses linked to poverty in less-affluent countries. These diseases are generally related to livestock or environmental sanitation. Rapid urbanization introduces factors (e.g., the intensification of production through cross-breeding with exotic cattle breeds) that increase the risk of zoonoses.

Public concern is driven by an understandable fear of unknown contagions, which can be escalated by media coverage and raise tremendous anxiety. This concern, however, does not necessarily reflect the actual burden or cost of disease. In less-affluent nations and countries in transition, the burden and cost of re-emerging and endemic zoonoses (with the exception of HIV) outweigh that of emerging zoonoses. Yet, re-emerging and endemic diseases attract much less attention and generate less political engagement than emerging diseases. For example, SARS and HPAI garnered much attention and were estimated to have cost billions of dollars, despite the fact that the actual burden of these diseases was quite small. Conversely, endemic diseases carry both a high cost and a high burden. Since countries that are unable to carry out early detection and rapid response represent a threat to all other countries, it is in the interest of all countries to contribute to global surveillance and control.

While factors influencing the emergence and persistence of zoonoses are more fully understood at the molecular level, there is much to be learned about the determinants of transmission at the population level in specific settings. Comparatively little is known about critical socioeconomic and ecological determinants of zoonoses. Research focuses mostly on the virulence of pathogens and the host-pathogen interaction at the individual level. But the population dynamics of human and animal hosts are equally important factors for transmission, and their effect on transmission may even supersede the virulence of a pathogen. Additionally, there is a lack of understanding regarding intervention effectiveness across all biological, environmental, social, and psychological determinants. Models have been developed that reveal the points of vulnerability where interventions against zoonoses will be most effective. Such models can direct the adaptation of policies to account for contextual social and ecological conditions, especially when economic considerations are integrated (Narrod, 2012).

Social and/or economic opportunities and challenges

Despite the wide use of the term One Health, it lacks a theoretical framework and a socioeconomic perspective. The recognition of inextricable linkages among human, livestock, companion animals, and wildlife is a necessary requirement for One Health; however, it is not sufficient. The success of One Health is dependent on the demonstration of an added value of health and well-being of humans and animals and/or financial savings from closer cooperation of human and animal health. In different African and Asian settings, we have applied and validated the concept of One Health, showing the highly synergistic benefits of a close interplay between human and animal health. For example, research in Mongolia shows that nationwide, mass vaccination of livestock to prevent human brucellosis would not be cost effective if the health sector had to pay for the full cost. However, if costs of livestock vaccination were shared by a variety of sectors (i.e., agricultural, public health, and private households) in proportion to their benefit, the intervention may be largely profitable for the health and agricultural sectors (Roth et al., 2003).

It is proposed that an opportunity exists to improve infectious disease control by building upon and extending the theory of intervention effectiveness to the animal-human interface. The effectiveness of an intervention (e.g., a drug or vaccine) — which is measured by the proportion of humans and/or animal populations covered, cured, or protected — may be much lower than its actual biological curative or preventive efficacy. A vaccine or drug's level of effectiveness is determined by factors including availability, accessibility, and affordability. Control programs need to be adequate and accepted in different sociocultural contexts, while simultaneously ensuring diagnostic accuracy, health care provider compliance, and consumer adherence. Figure 1 presents a hypothetical example of a drug or vaccine that has an efficacy of 100%, yet a final effectiveness of only 15% at the community level. Even if all influencing factors have a relatively high individual performance, this multiplicative effect means that interventions may drop below the threshold coverage necessary to interrupt transmission of a zoonotic disease. A combination of quantitative and qualitative epidemiological, social, and anthropological methods will enable identification of the most sensitive determinants of intervention effectiveness (Zinsstag et al., 2011). Determinants of the effectiveness of surveillance and interventions at different scales, ranging from the household to the government level, can then be connected by epidemiological, sociocultural, and economic studies to build a comprehensive and quantifiable One Health effectiveness framework that provides convincing evidence for policy and practice.

Policy Issues

- To foster One Health, no new institutions or disciplines are needed. What is necessary is simply working together better within the existing institutions. Otherwise, the added value is lost due to additional costs.

- The International tripartite of the World Health Organization (WHO), the Food and Agriculture Organization (FAO), and the World Organisation for Animal Health (OIE) should lead the technical aspects of One Health, while the World Bank should be the leader in One Health's economic domain. The OIE Performance of Veterinary Services and WHO international health regulations tools should be joined together. At the governmental level, national or provincial authorities should develop decentralized One Health leadership.

- When assessing the effectiveness of One Health approaches, which aim to foster closer cooperation between human and animal health, it is important to measure their success in saving financial resources and improving human and animal health. Further research is needed to strengthen this evidence involving social science, economics, and ecology.

- The effectiveness of locally adapted infectious disease surveillance, prevention, and elimination strategies depends on a greater commitment through transdisciplinary, participatory stakeholder processes which involve authorities, communities, and experts.

- The private sector should be encouraged to engage in public-private partnerships to control and eliminate zoonoses in less-affluent countries (e.g., dairy industry to engage in brucellosis control).

- One Health curricula for medical and veterinary faculties are needed to prepare a new generation of highly competent cross-sector networkers to mainstream One Health.

References

Narrod, C., Zinsstag, J., Tiongco, M. (2012). A One Health framework for estimating the economic costs of zoonotic diseases on society. *EcoHealth,* in press.

Roth, F., Zinsstag, J., Orkhon, D., Chimed-Ochir, G., Hutton, G., Cosivi, O., Carrin, G., Otte, J. (2003). Human health benefits from livestock vaccination for brucellosis: Case study. *Bulletin of the World Health Organization, 81,* 867–876.

Zinsstag J., Bonfoh, B., Cissé, G., Nguyen, V.H., Silué, B., N'Guessan, T.S., ... Tanner, M. (2011). Towards equity effectiveness in health interventions. *In:* Weismann, U., Hurni, H., editors. *Research for Sustainable Development: Foundations, Experiences, and Perspectives.* Perspectives of the Swiss National Centre of Competence in Research (NCCR) North-South, Geographica Bernensis, Berne, Switzerland, 6, 623–640.

*** A policy position paper prepared for presentation at the conference on Emerging and Persistent Infectious Diseases (EPID): Focus on the Societal and Economic Context, convened by the Institute on Science for Global Policy (ISGP) July 8–11, 2012, at George Mason University, Fairfax, Virginia.*

Figure 1.
From efficacy to community effectiveness of an intervention. Adapted from "From 'one medicine' to 'one health' and systemic approaches to health and well-being," by Zinsstag, J., Schelling, E., Waltner-Toews, D., Tanner, M., 2011, *Preventive Veterinary Medicine*, 101, 148–156. Adapted with permission.

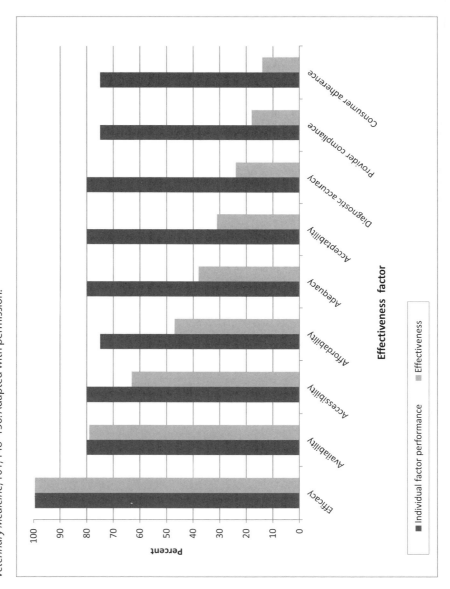

Debate Summary

The following summary is based on notes recorded by the ISGP staff during the not-for-attribution debate of the policy position paper prepared by Prof. Jakob Zinsstag (see above). Prof. Zinsstag initiated the debate with a 5-minute statement of his views and then actively engaged the conference participants, including other authors, throughout the remainder of the 90-minute period. This Debate Summary represents the ISGP's best effort to accurately capture the comments offered and questions posed by all participants, as well as those responses made by Prof. Zinsstag. Given the not-for-attribution format of the debate, the views comprising this summary do not necessarily represent the views of Prof. Zinsstag, as evidenced by his policy position paper. Rather, it is, and should be read as, an overview of the areas of agreement and disagreement that emerged from all those participating in the critical debate.

Debate conclusions

- Clear linkages among human, animal (domestic and wild), and environmental health frequently impact the emergence, persistence, and spread of infectious diseases in human populations. Yet the various sectors that are charged with protecting each of these arenas are commonly segregated in mission and scope of work.

- Multidisciplinary collaborations are critical to control infectious diseases that are zoonotic or have environmental origins, as well as to ensure that societal and/or economic considerations are appropriately factored into disease prevention and mitigation efforts. There is a strong need to amplify multidisciplinary collaborations (e.g., cross-sector linkages) in advance of crises. These efforts begin with improving trust and partnerships across the diverse groups charged with infectious disease control (e.g., nongovernmental organizations [NGOs], national and local governments, public health agencies, and scientists). Rewards for joint initiatives may help bridge the gap between various sectors.

- The One Health approach is a valuable *framework* for determining where it is cost-effective to jointly address infectious disease problems across sectors and to bolster collaborations across stakeholders that frequently function in siloed disciplines. No new One Health institutions should be created for this purpose; rather, a bottom-up approach within existing intergovernmental agencies, national and local governments, and other relevant groups should be implemented to capitalize on One Health principles where appropriate.

- The local level should be considered as a fruitful starting place for the implementation of One Health concepts and for setting priorities associated with the control of infectious diseases. In the international arena, the tripartite of the World Health Organization (WHO), the Food and Agriculture Organization (FAO), and the World Organisation for Animal Health (OIE) should be further empowered to take the lead on One Health efforts, including setting standards. For One Health initiatives to increasingly receive a portion of the limited resources available at any level, more evidence-based research will be needed to demonstrate the economic value of specific cross-sector collaborations and interventions.

- Capacity building in less-affluent regions is particularly important for infectious disease surveillance initiatives. While capacity building related to other aspects of infectious disease control (e.g., laboratories and training) may also hold great value, it is critical for such initiatives to be structured in ways that foster sustainability within the areas receiving assistance.

Current realities

Multidisciplinary collaboration — across human, animal, and environmental sectors — was widely viewed as critically important for the effective control of infectious diseases. While it was generally agreed that multidisciplinary efforts do currently occur, divergent opinions were expressed regarding the extent to which different sectors (e.g., human and animal) presently work together and the degree to which further collaboration should be required (e.g., via One Health).

Discord stemming from disparate opinions on the definition and purpose of One Health highlighted that the value of One Health, particularly for infectious disease control, is currently undergoing significant scrutiny. The underlying principles of One Health as a concept that is focused on drawing attention to the inextricable linkages among human, animal (domestic and wild), and ecosystem health were generally accepted. While such linkages were deemed vital to the prevention and mitigation of infectious diseases, questions were raised regarding whether the goals of One Health are significantly different from multidisciplinary collaboration and how One Health can be practically implemented.

The protection of human health has largely been the main priority of the infectious disease control initiatives promoted within national governments.

Consequently, unless a specific connection to human health has been demonstrated, animal and environmental health issues have frequently received less attention and fewer resources.

It was acknowledged that human and animal health sectors are mostly segregated within both governmental and intergovernmental agencies and that, although they do periodically work together, collaborations most commonly occur during times of crisis (e.g., during the European bovine spongiform encephalopathy crisis that began in the late 20th century and the 2009 "swine flu" pandemic [PDM 2009 H1N1]).

Fragmentation of responsibilities among the NGOs, national and local governments, public health agencies, and scientists charged with infectious disease control has led to duplication of efforts across and within human, animal, and environmental sectors. Such duplication has, in turn, given rise to increased costs. It was asserted that fragmentation predominantly occurs when leadership on specific issues has not been clearly identified.

The reality that human, animal, and environmental linkages have serious implications for ensuring human health was highlighted by anecdotal evidence, including observations that infectious diseases are more likely to jump the species barrier when humans encroach on animal habitats. This scenario has given rise to increased pandemic potential. While integrated studies that examine the human-animal interface using nonreductionist methods until recently have been largely absent from scientific research, it was noted that interest in this investigative area is gradually expanding.

It was widely recognized that more-affluent countries focus their attention on the control of emerging zoonotic diseases even though persistent zoonotic diseases pose significantly greater problems in less-wealthy areas such as in Africa and Asia. Many persistent diseases have been labeled as "neglected diseases" that continually burden neglected communities.

Social and/or economic opportunities and challenges

While it was argued that moving from a sectoral to a societal perspective (i.e., considering the public good as a whole) has positive human health implications, it was also noted that the present siloization of departments and agencies creates barriers that are challenging to overcome. For example, ministers of agriculture have a different set of priorities than ministers of health and it can be difficult to get these two groups to work together outside of their traditional purviews, particularly when one side does not perceive there to be an economic benefit related to their specific mission.

Attention was drawn to the potential for infectious disease control to be more efficiently and cost-effectively undertaken by proactively seeking solutions that jointly address animal and human health problems. This was illustrated by a successful intervention effort that simultaneously vaccinated cattle, women, and children in parts of Sahelian Africa where livestock vaccination was more common than human vaccination. The intervention significantly raised vaccination rates in humans and, at the same time, saved approximately 15% in costs through the sharing of transport and culture costs among veterinarians, public health personnel, and nurses.

Traditional approaches to the amelioration of diseases affecting human health focus largely on humans themselves. Yet, it was demonstrated that shifting attention toward disease control in animals can elicit improvements in human health for certain zoonotic infectious diseases. This was illustrated by the case of rabies where intervening in humans (e.g., via vaccinations) is less effective than intervening in the animal reservoir because, in the former, animal-to-human transmission is not interrupted. In addition to reducing the prevalence of disease among humans, studies have shown that rabies vaccinations in dog populations are initially more costly, but have a higher long-term return on investment.

Decisions related to funding are not generally made at the macro long-term level. Therefore it has been difficult to translate aggregate societal benefit into action when not all of the sectors can be ensured that they will actually see benefits to justify their investments. For instance, the time scale for establishing benefits may be longer than their budget cycles and/or another sector may gain disproportionately from the initial investment.

Efforts to improve societal human health related to infectious diseases are frequently stymied by economic considerations at the individual level, as demonstrated by the ongoing issue of antibiotic resistance. While the overuse of antibiotics in animal populations has substantially contributed to antibiotic resistance in humans, livestock farmers continue to use antibiotics because they improve production. It was suggested that banning the use of common antibiotics in animals would rectify this problem. This proposal was contested by those who felt that the livestock community is too politically strong for this to be a realistic option.

Questions were raised regarding whether it is in the interest of more-wealthy countries to intervene in less-wealthy countries for the control of endemic diseases. From a cost-benefit perspective, it is not economically rational for the United States and Europe to treat and control many endemic diseases outside their borders. While it was suggested that improving the capacity of less-affluent areas to manage endemic diseases may also ensure that the necessary capacity is in place should an emerging disease appear, many felt that the onus should not fall on affluent regions. They reasoned that interventions by outside agencies may be viewed as subsidies that can eventually become entitlements that produce distortions in a country's overall health.

There was some discussion on whether creating One Health courses in veterinary, medical, and public health curricula would help train a younger generation to view infectious disease control more holistically. Although it was believed that such courses would help engender greater trust between younger individuals within these communities, it was also felt that the utility of such courses may be limited by the present lack of reward mechanisms for multidisciplinary careers and research.

Some concern was expressed that the One Health approach is an advocacy mechanism for veterinarians to improve their social standing and increase their resources. Although many disagreed with this view, it was maintained that the burden falls on One Health supporters to prove the value of their ideals for infectious disease control.

Policy issues

The view that the One Health approach needs to be considered as a *framework* through which infectious disease control efforts should be assessed and implemented garnered much support. There was general consensus that no new institutions should be created for the express purpose of facilitating the implementation of One Health principles. It was strongly contended that significantly improving cross-sector collaboration through a bottom-up approach within existing intergovernmental agencies, national and local governments, and other stakeholders would be the most successful route toward capitalizing on the inherent linkages among human, animal, and environmental health.

The local level was believed to be a fruitful starting point for practically implementing One Health concepts. Integrated social, cultural, and ecological assessments were pinpointed as valuable tools that should be used for identifying community-based priorities and contextualized interventions within local settings. Additionally, it was asserted that efforts should be made to determine where local cross-sector solutions to infectious disease problems can improve the cost-effectiveness of interventions.

In the international arena, it was recommended that the tripartite of WHO, FAO, and OIE continue to take the lead in fostering collaborations and setting standards. To improve the tripartite's effectiveness, it was asserted that these intergovernmental agencies should be further empowered to look beyond their traditional purviews, particularly within collaborative settings. The smallest of these agencies, OIE, may require additional financial support, but it was not determined whether this is indeed the case or how much assistance would be required. In terms of standards, it was urged that efforts should be made to improve adherence to the WHO International Health Regulations (IHR) and to increase adoption of the OIE Tool for the Evaluation of Performance of Veterinary Services (PVS).

Improving the implementation of the concepts underlying One Health was deemed essential. Within this effort, proactively raising the level of trust across sectors was considered especially critical. Attention was called to PDM 2009 H1N1 to illustrate why it is imperative for human and animal health communities to have sound relationships before a crisis occurs. This includes making sure that mutual respect and partnerships are already in place. It was asserted that the steps necessary to enhance trust include building bridges among stakeholders (e.g., ministers in different governmental sectors, NGOs, scientists, and the public); sharing data and samples; and the promotion of cost sharing where economical.

It was argued that changing mindsets in a world where human, animal, and environmental health communities not only have a long history of siloization, but also are frequently motivated to remain siloed (e.g., via separate funding streams) requires new incentives to build linkages across sectors. Rewarding cross-sector relationships in ways that are economically and professionally profitable was suggested as a critical step toward bolstering multidisciplinary collaboration.

It was widely acknowledged that funding priorities for the prevention and mitigation of infectious diseases are heavily based on where the greatest return on investment can be achieved. For One Health initiatives to receive a larger portion of the limited resources available, more evidence-based research will be needed to demonstrate the economic value of specific cross-sector collaborations and interventions. Data sharing across disciplines was considered an integral component of such research so that models and analyses can be created that accurately reflect the connection between risk factors within all relevant health spheres. Additionally, for funding to be justified, it was urged that sensitivity analyses should be conducted to help demonstrate why resources should be targeted to a particular geographic area or topic versus other needs.

Further incorporation of sociocultural and economic factors into multidisciplinary infectious disease control efforts (e.g., research and implementation) was recommended as an important way to strengthen the effectiveness of such activities. Gaining a greater understanding of the societal underpinnings of where and why diseases emerge and persist, as well as the economics that are associated with disease proliferation, was strongly supported.

Capacity building in less-wealthy countries was urged as a way to improve infectious disease control from within the most affected geographic areas. While it was agreed that there is a global advantage to more-affluent regions helping their less-wealthy counterparts enhance their surveillance capacity (e.g., to improve awareness of the emergence of new diseases or transmission that could reach more-wealthy areas), some felt that caution should be exercised in other forms of capacity-building assistance that could lead to entitlements. As such, it was recommended that nonsurveillance related capacity building should focus on activities that will eventually be sustainable by the countries receiving assistance.

Solving Food Safety Problems Without Antiquated Regulation and Inspection**

Richard Williams, Ph.D., M.A.
Director of Policy Research, Mercatus Center, George Mason University,
Arlington, Virginia

Summary

The United States system of ensuring food safety is more than 100 years old and, until very recently, was the primary system designed to ensure food safety. The system assumes that primarily federal regulators have the necessary knowledge to instruct food manufacturers on producing safe food, with both federal and state governments enforcing their respective regulations. While there have been notable successes in the last century — such as mandatory pasteurization for milk and other products, low acid canned food rules, and basic sanitation requirements — much of this progress was achieved in the first half of the 20th century. In the last 30 years, the incidence of foodborne disease has changed very little.

Achieving a safer food supply requires a redefinition of the role of the public sector that takes advantage of new technologies. Traditionally, consumers have been forced to rely on government regulation and inspection because private manufacturers were rarely held accountable for problems. Even when contaminated foods were traced back to negligent manufacturers, outside of large national outbreaks, there was little chance that news about it would be widespread. Today, there are systems in place, based on new technology, that are becoming increasingly better at tracking food safety problems to individual production plants. With this technology, we can provide producers with incentives to prevent food safety problems from occurring in the first place, taking advantage of their comparative advantages. This represents a tremendous improvement over reliance on regulation and inspection and suggests that more progress can be made by improving these traceback systems.

Current realities

The food industry is growing both in the number of firms (more than one million manufacturing and retail) and in the wide variety of technologies used to produce foods. These two developments make it extremely difficult for government agencies to: (i) have sufficient knowledge of the wide variety and continually changing mix of foods, packaging, and processes in individual plants to produce effective regulations and (ii) access sufficient resources to inspect firms often enough to ensure compliance. Because of this growth in complexity in food manufacturing, the Food and Drug Administration (FDA) in particular finds it increasingly difficult to have the necessary knowledge to meaningfully regulate food processing and packaging. On average, the FDA inspects firms about once every five years and samples only about 1% to 2% of all imported food products. In addition, the FDA often must react to political realities; rather than focus on protecting consumers, many regulations are formulated at the behest of one part of the industry to put another part of the industry at a competitive disadvantage.

With the advent of better traceback mechanisms and DNA fingerprinting that links pathogens from infected production plants to pathogens in food, the food industry has become more proactive in preventing food safety problems as they are becoming more accountable for disease outbreaks. In the past, when companies were the source of a foodborne disease outbreak, they faced only a slight chance of being identified as the origin of that outbreak. Now, the probability of being identified as responsible for a disease outbreak is greater than 50%. In addition, the growth of the Internet has ensured that essentially every outbreak is publicly reported nationally (many by private information suppliers). These developments have caused private food safety contracts to surface at every level, usually with the resultant increase in inspections. Final product manufacturers inspect ingredient suppliers, and, in turn, are inspected by supermarkets. All kinds of food manufacturers are inspected by insurance agents. In some cases, firms report weekly inspections. This has nothing to do with regulation, but rather with firms acting to prevent lawsuits, loss of sales, and recall costs.

Social and/or economic opportunities and challenges

Rather than being governed primarily by regulation, food manufacturers are increasingly governed by millions of contracts that are negotiated between food manufacturers and those they sell to (or that insure them), both domestically and internationally. These contracts cover specific conditions of food production and distribution and are written specifically for the type of product and package produced. When new information (e.g., root causes of outbreaks) is made available to the market, these private contracts change much more quickly and accurately than government regulations. Private inspections take place on a more frequent basis than even a combination of federal and state regulators could achieve with a realistic amount of public resources. In addition, thousands of new private food safety firms are now providing food manufacturers with both expert advice and third-party inspections. This new system will not eliminate all foodborne disease — pathogens are ubiquitous; new foods, equipment, and technologies are evolving — but constant and continuous monitoring can reduce illness.

The next major improvements in food safety are likely to come from new technologies or the broader acceptance of older technologies. Of the older technologies, irradiation has been proven safe but still faces an uphill battle for consumer acceptance given the public's poor understanding of the science behind it. Newer technologies, such as nanotechnology and the genetic modification of foods, hold promise for improvement, but are also subject to misunderstanding about the actual associated risks. Progress in these areas is hindered when people continue to treat new technologies as different simply because they are new, and thus think that they require precautions far greater than those given to existing technologies.

The biggest problem, however, is the misconception that the federal government is the sole source of assurance of safe food. Within the last few years, Congress has passed legislation much like the system of regulation and inspection developed for food safety at the turn of the 20th century. Instead of developing and complementing systems that hold firms accountable for problems *ex post* (i.e., after the fact), government remains fixated with a more *ex ante* (i.e., before an event) approach: "command and control." These systems are "comfortable" for incumbent industries that routinely lobby for more regulation and larger budgets for the agencies. As a result, new regulations pile on top of old ones. The government has no ability to enforce them, yet regulations give consumers the illusion of control. The system is also increasingly reflected in the international arena where the same problems (lack of knowledge and inspectional capacity) persist. While there have been encouraging movements toward risk-based systems, these systems are being used to support more federal regulations rather than feeding information to the private sector to make the private contracts discussed above more effective.

The primary challenge is to rethink the role of the FDA, an organization that is more than 100 years old and has never had to rethink its basic mission.

Policy issues

- Federal resources (both U.S. and other national governments) should be reallocated for developing better traceback technologies, including the development and use of such technologies as radio frequency identification tags (RFIDs) and bar codes that travel throughout the production process. Governments should focus fewer resources on plant-by-plant inspections, but more on enlarging government DNA fingerprinting libraries, both domestically and internationally, as well as developing better fingerprinting tools such as pulsed field gel electrophoresis (PFGE). These libraries should be open to the public.

- In general, food safety agencies should end most command and control regulations unless there is strong evidence of effective solutions that pass a strict benefit-cost test. Instead, these food safety agencies should work to understand the private sector system of contracts and inspection and identify any holes in the system. In addition, more resources should be devoted to the production and public distribution of information on food safety, such as the identification of root causes of outbreaks. This should include the location in the system of the problems among producers, retailers, and consumers, and producing risk assessments and benefit-cost analyses assessing problems and potential solutions for food safety problems. The latter part of this recommendation supports the Actionable Next Step on information sharing that has emerged from prior ISGP conferences. However, it should be expanded to include the private sector.

- The federal government should ensure that all new food safety technologies are evaluated in a risk/benefit framework. High priority (i.e., speedy development) should be given to those technologies that hold the most promise for enhancing food safety. Faster federal government approval processes for new technologies should be developed using risk/benefit methodologies. New technologies should be treated on the same risk basis as existing technologies. Overcoming the obstacles to risk/benefit approval of new technologies will require the focused use of risk communication techniques that have developed over the last several decades.

- The primary obstacle to a new focus on market accountability is federal policy makers' lack of knowledge of the current actual system that governs food safety. In addition, strong opposition is likely to come from incumbent industry members who benefit from the system as well as from those who prefer government command and control for political reasons. Overcoming these obstacles will require research into the private system of contracts and inspections as they are developing. It will also require education in the academic community and for policy makers by both government and academic researchers. This implies that greater government oversight and more standards — as stated in the Actionable Next Steps on food safety and security — are not likely to be productive.

References

Williams, R. A. (2010, November). *A new role for the FDA in food safety* (Working Paper 10–69). Arlington, VA: Mercatus Center at George Mason University.

Henson, S., & Humphrey, J. (2009). *The impacts of private food safety standards on the food chain and on public standard setting processes.* Joint FAO/WHO Food Standards Programme, Codex Alimentarius Commission, 32nd Session.

*** A policy position paper prepared for presentation at the conference on Emerging and Persistent Infectious Diseases (EPID): Focus on the Societal and Economic Context, convened by the Institute on Science for Global Policy (ISGP) July 8–11, 2012, at George Mason University, Fairfax, Virginia.*

Debate Summary

The following summary is based on notes recorded by the ISGP staff during the not-for-attribution debate of the policy position paper prepared by Dr. Richard Williams (see above). Dr. Williams initiated the debate with a 5-minute statement of his views and then actively engaged the conference participants, including other authors, throughout the remainder of the 90-minute period. This Debate Summary represents the ISGP's best effort to accurately capture the comments offered and questions posed by all participants, as well as those responses made by Dr. Williams. Given the not-for-attribution format of the debate, the views comprising this summary do not necessarily represent the views of Dr. Williams, as evidenced by his policy position paper. Rather, it is, and should be read as, an overview of the areas of agreement and disagreement that emerged from all those participating in the critical debate.

Debate conclusions

- While it was agreed that the government should play a major role in ensuring that food is safe, there was disagreement about whether the focus of governmental efforts should be on regulation and inspection, or whether emphasis should shift toward incentivizing companies to voluntarily self-regulate through methods such as enhanced traceback technology, as well as research and education.

- The continued emphasis on increased regulations and inspections as the United States government's primary method of preventing foodborne illness outbreaks has both benefits and challenges as viewed through the focused and/or proprietary interests of government regulators, food companies, and consumers. Since under current circumstances, the U.S. Food and Drug Administration (FDA) has limited capacity for implementing such ongoing inspections of domestic firms and imported foods, the effectiveness of government regulation and inspections needs to be better evaluated.

• Globally, there has been a tremendous increase in self-regulation through private food safety contracts. The benefits of self-regulation via private contracts versus government regulations include the ability to (i) implement tailored solutions and (ii) rapidly change procedures based on the latest research. The potential negative consequences of privatizing food safety include the loss of domestic and international consumer confidence in the safety of the food supply and thus a retrenchment in the general commitment to ensure public welfare is a priority.

• Since the continued development of enhanced traceback technologies is increasing the likelihood that a private company will be identified as the source of an outbreak, the continuation of efforts to improve these technologies is critical. It remains unclear whether the best venues for the development of traceback technology are in the government, the private sector, or public-private partnerships. Improvements in traceback technologies can lead to safer foods by promoting self-regulation, since it places the incentive for food safety on the producer.

Current realities

Concerns over current food safety are present both in the U.S. and internationally, especially in government agencies. There was a general consensus that serious food safety problems exist and that little progress to address them has been made over the past 30 years. It was asserted that within the U.S., the primary method of preventing outbreaks supported by the federal government is the continued emphasis on increased regulations and inspections.

It was agreed that the number of new food safety regulations is increasing. For example, the Food Safety Modernization Act (FSMA) has called for approximately 15 new regulations and more government inspectors. The current "command and control" system has been designed such that outbreaks are followed by congressional hearings that traditionally lead to the passage of new laws, which subsequently lead to new FDA regulations. It was emphasized that the current regulatory system of food safety consists of government oversight of inspections.

It was recognized that the FDA does not currently have the capacity to implement ongoing inspections on all domestic firms, and only inspects U.S. companies once every five to 10 years. It was also noted that the FDA only samples approximately 1% to 2% of all imported foods.

The status quo of continually increasing government regulations and inspections has received widespread support and is perpetuated through support from several types of vested interests. First, large food companies support the continued implementation of new regulations since such "command and control" regulations impose fixed costs on smaller competitors. This provides a competitive advantage for large food companies since the added expenses of meeting regulations serve as a barrier to market entry for smaller companies. It was countered, however, that businesses do not necessarily favor additional regulations, but do support effective food safety regulations because any food safety failure hurts all companies.

Second, it was argued that government interests perpetuate the system of increased regulations. Regulations are often implemented solely to meet export requirements, even when their effectiveness is in question. It was also stated that some government workers feel their jobs are threatened by the increase and effectiveness of private inspections. Further, it was suggested that for many individuals in the Senior Executive Service of the government, the passing of new regulations is viewed positively. The view that government regulatory agencies create regulations primarily because it generates more work was strongly disputed. It was recognized that the FDA is under tremendous pressure to effectively regulate food safety through a wide range of entities including the food industry and nonprofit organizations. The FDA is, of course, required to do so once Congress passes a law.

Third, it was noted that laws and regulations are often reactionary, created in response to consumer pressure that occurs immediately after an outbreak. These command and control regulations, established after an outbreak, were said to bolster consumer confidence in food safety.

Over the past 10 to 20 years, new and improved traceback technologies have been developed including DNA fingerprinting that can match a contaminated person to a plant and radio frequency identification tags for foods. It was estimated that more than half of all foodborne outbreaks can now be traced to a processing plant, and it was agreed that developing such technologies will continue to enhance domestic and international traceback. The increased likelihood of being identified as the source of an outbreak was said to act as a deterrent to would-be offenders.

Because each entity wants to avoid being connected to a disease outbreak, there has been a significant increase in private food safety contracts worldwide at all stages in the food supply chain. These efforts include third-party inspectors and private inspections. For example, insurance agencies are establishing their own food safety contracts and conducting their own inspections. Many food safety private contracts were said to go well beyond standards set by the FDA or the U.S. Department of Agriculture (USDA). It was asserted that in private markets, some firms are being inspected at least once a year, or even once a week, and that the federal government is unaware of the level of private contracts that exist.

Social and/or economic opportunities and challenges

There was disagreement about the effectiveness of increased government and self-regulation on food safety, especially since governments rarely evaluate the effectiveness of their regulations. There was agreement that progress has been minimal over the past 30 years in terms of food safety. While this lack of progress may show the ineffectiveness of regulations in the last 20 to 30 years, it was noted that even though self-regulation (through private food safety contracts) is increasing, food safety is not improving. Thus, it was argued that the rise of private contracts has not been noticeably effective either. It was conceded that more evidence is needed to more clearly demonstrate whether either self-regulation or private contracts have been effective.

The effectiveness of Hazard Analysis and Critical Control Points (HAACP) was also questioned. The USDA, for example, requires prevention and has been operating under HAACP non-"command and control" since 1996. Doubts were raised whether USDA's HAACP program has accomplished results close to those initially predicted, namely that it would prevent 80% of all foodborne diseases. It was contended that benefits of implementing HAACP actually came from the HAACP prerequisite program which made the meat and poultry plants cleaner.

The ability of traceback methods to identify the source of a foodborne illness outbreak was debated. While the promise of current and new technology was touted, it was agreed that traceback itself can be very complicated and sometimes ineffective in identifying an outbreak's source. The use of traceback was said to be especially complicated for use with imported foods. Traceback technology in Europe was believed to be more advanced than in the United States, although it was said that the U.S. is more advanced than Europe in terms of PulseNet.

It was agreed that food safety technologies are advancing rapidly and that the continuous monitoring of factories and grocery stores may be possible soon. However, it was asserted that technologies, even when effective, are not always embraced for a variety of reasons. Irradiation, for example, was identified as being "one of the major public health failures in the U.S.", due to initially being understood as "nuclear radiation". Such labeling discouraged public acceptance based on the incorrect view that the radiation used was at a dangerous level. Better communication is required to counter such misinformation about such a technology where the health risk is in reality minimal at worst.

It was also agreed that much research remains to be done to determine what level of pathogens cause a disease outbreak. It was agreed that what may be safe for one person may not be safe for someone else. For example, although research indicates that 100,000 units of listeria is the minimum infectious dose, a smaller dose may result in poisoning among highly sensitive people. As a consequence, the FDA states that any amount of listeria exposure may be unsafe.

It was widely agreed that consumer behavior plays a large role in food safety. An example was provided whereby in one country, people wash their fruits and vegetables in a dilute of Clorox solution; these same fruits and vegetables are imported to the U.S. where many people rinse them or do not wash them at all.

Policy issues

The role of the U.S. federal government in food safety was debated. While it was agreed that the government should play a major role in ensuring that food is safe, there was disagreement about whether the focus should be on regulation and inspection, or whether emphasis should shift toward incentivizing companies to voluntarily self-regulate through methods such as enhanced traceback technology, as well as research and education.

While it was agreed that in the past, FDA regulations such as mandating pasteurization were necessary and effective, there was disagreement about the current relevance of government regulations and inspection. While government regulations and inspection were viewed as necessary for food safety efforts, some food companies incorrectly believe that preventive food safety measures cost more than mitigating outbreaks and conducting recalls. From this perspective, these companies may not be incentivized to implement food safety activities without government regulations and inspections. It was also agreed that government inspection is especially necessary for imported food and products where history has demonstrated that the sequestration and removal of some imported food by the FDA have prevented the public from being exposed to potentially dangerous foods.

However, the current system of government regulations and inspections was viewed as not working well enough for a number of reasons. For example, one agency cannot effectively regulate all firms because of the wide variety in foods, packaging, transportation, and farm-to-farm differences that determine what is safe food. It was recognized that the FDA has limited capacity to implement ongoing inspections on all domestic or imported foods. Government regulation was thought by some to undermine technological advancement in food safety because companies may not be incentivized to improve beyond minimum standards. In addition, it was argued that federal regulations, which can take years to pass, may be obsolete by the time they are put into place.

From one perspective, the resources currently used for regulation and inspection should be shifted to improve traceback technology such as DNA fingerprinting and enhancing the PulseNet lab. A government focus on enhanced traceback would lead to safer foods by placing the incentive for food safety on the producer, which would result in increased voluntary self-regulation. With enhanced traceback, a plant that is the source of a disease outbreak may be properly identified and subjected to penalties and additional costs, including financial losses (the loss of food, recall costs, loss of sales), and/or a loss of reputation or brand. Such a plant might even be banned from producing food for human consumption. It was questioned, however, whether penalties would be significant enough to inspire a change from a federal to industry-based system of food safety since insurance companies would bear the burden of costs of an outbreak.

It was also suggested that improved traceback would increase the safety of imports to the U.S. Countries with repeated violations might be placed on automatic detention, which may encourage them to improve their food safety efforts. Enhanced traceback could be even more effective in incentivizing self-regulation in the current age of the Internet, whereby the manufacturer at the source of a foodborne illness outbreak is rapidly known to the public.

It was agreed that the effectiveness of traceback in promoting self-regulation is complicated by "gaming," whereby parent companies may create shell companies that have no assets. If an outbreak is traced to such a shell company, it could go bankrupt without impacting the financial health of the parent company. Self-regulation might address this issue since more supermarkets are privately contracting the responsibility for food safety and therefore, are less likely to accept food from a shell company.

There was disagreement about whose role it is to develop better traceback technology. While government resources might be allocated for the development and implementation of traceback technology, the development of the traceback technology itself could be conducted in the private sector or through public-private partnerships. The distribution of these responsibilities remained unresolved.

It was suggested that voluntary self-regulation through private sector contracts represents a vast improvement over government regulations. Those with knowledge of particular farms are better able to identify tailored solutions that are more effective than one-size-fits-all approaches. The private sector is also able to rapidly adapt its efforts to the latest research. Government agencies can gain a clearer understanding of the current systems used by the private sector designed to eliminate redundancy and effectively fill gaps.

Potentially negative consequences of privatizing food safety were noted, including the loss in consumer confidence both domestically and internationally. Concern was expressed that countries outside the U.S. could use the existence of a privatized system as a trade barrier to U.S. exports. It was countered, however, that many consumers are not even aware of regulations, and that they do not make consumers feel safer. Food companies often do not have a market incentive to defend the country, and it was questioned whether encouraging self-regulation for food safety would be effective in the food security arena, (i.e., protection against deliberate attack). While a strategy centered on traceback and PulseNet was criticized for its narrow focus on reaction and not prevention, it was recognized that traceback is a prevention strategy and that food companies implement food safety practices based on their fear of being at the source of an outbreak.

The federal government's role in research and education was discussed. It was maintained that food safety efforts should include basic research on the root causes of foodborne disease. There was a call for education, training, and more appropriate messaging in terms of food safety (e.g., successes and failures) to industry, government, and consumers. It would be productive to emphasize information on proper nutrition and the safe handling of food into the elementary school curriculum. It was agreed that consumer expectations of food safety are unrealistic, and that consumers must learn that food will never be 100% safe. Educational efforts were expected to limit consumers' appeals for the creation of new laws and regulations with each outbreak. Education could also play a key role in motivating government agencies to shift funding from regulation and inspection toward more preventive efforts.

The importance of public-private partnerships in food safety efforts was highlighted. Partnerships in the pharmaceutical world, whereby companies and the government have worked together to develop agreements that have addressed companies' issues with regulation and government need for certain drugs, were provided as an example of success.

Translating Technical Advances in Genomics to the Developing World: Addressing Cultural Needs as Part of Policy-Making**

Vanessa M. Hayes, Ph.D.
Professor of Genomic Medicine, J. Craig Venter Institute, San Diego, CA
Honorary Professor of Medical Sciences, University of Limpopo,
Limpopo Province, South Africa

Summary

Technical and computational advances in generating and deciphering the DNA code of living organisms (including the human genome and microbiome) have revolutionized medical research efforts, including those targeting emerging and persistent infectious diseases (EPID). However, these efforts have largely targeted the world outside of Africa. Africa, the continent with the largest genomic, linguistic, cultural, and EPID diversity, is only now seeing the first signs of these advances. Major limitations to accessing genomics consist of social (including cultural) and economic factors. The world outside of Africa needs to address the significant role Africa has played and continues to play in shaping the globe, from our human origins to the large biodiversity that has led to a number of EPID outbreaks. The societal and economic challenges that face all 54 African countries calls for a concerted effort from the international community. Building bridges between non-African and African countries, where communication and flow of technology and information is unidirectional, is the ultimate way that Africa can embrace western technology and that non-African countries can embrace African culture. This paper will address why the western world needs to embrace African culture to be successful in translating technical advances in genomics within the region.

Current realities

Technical advances in DNA sequencing and computational analysis have revolutionized health care and created an era of "genomic medicine." In brief, genomic medicine is the use of information from the genome (e.g., the complete DNA sequence of a human and/or pathogen) to guide clinical management. The draft sequence of the Human Genome (completed 10 years ago) provided a reference to capture DNA variation essential to defining disease susceptibility or resistance, disease outcomes, or response to treatments. The human host is, however, more than just its cells and DNA; microbial cells outnumber human cells by a factor of 10 to 1 in any healthy adult. Since extensive human microbial diversity will also impact health status in infectious diseases, genomics, within the context of this paper, may cover the human genome (host) and/or the human microbiome (pathogen). The current reality is that while the benefits of genomics are widespread in the western world, the regions where EPID often arise and reach epidemic levels have largely been excluded from the genomics revolution.

Africa is the second largest continent, home to one-sixth of the world's population and approximately 2,000 linguistic groups (representing almost as many cultures). According to the World Health Organization (WHO), Africa is home to the highest recorded mortality rates for the top three infectious diseases: malaria, tuberculosis (TB), and HIV/AIDS. The United Nations Children's Fund (UNICEF) and WHO have noted some sobering realities, including that malaria claims the life of a child in Africa every 30 seconds, in 2010 more than 270 cases of TB per 100,000 population was recorded for sub-Saharan Africa, and by 2010 an estimated 15.7 million children in sub-Saharan Africa had lost at least one parent to AIDS. As stated in the Areas of Consensus that emerged from prior ISGP conferences, there is no doubt that the potential for one of Emerging and Persistent Infectious Diseases (EPID) to reach pandemic levels is inevitable. Thus, the question is whether the Actionable Next Steps to prevent such a major global threat are adequate for the African context? Africa needs to be included in the revolution of genomic medicine. Is Africa ready for this revolution or are we, as scientists and policy makers, ready to accept the challenges of making the genomic revolution work for — and not against — Africa? This paper addresses challenges associated with the acquisition, sharing, and implementation of genomic data of relevance to EPID based on diverse cultural and economic systems of relevance within Africa.

Social and/or economic opportunities and challenges

Why is African culture so important? African culture is the very essence of life itself. To quote Dr. Maulana Karenga, chair of the Department of Africana Studies at California State University, Long Beach, "Culture is the totality of thought and practice by which a people creates itself, celebrates, sustains and develops itself and introduces itself to history and humanity (Karenga, 2009)." One must caution the western world that it is ignorant to interpret African culture as "backward." A Senegal proverb states: "The chameleon changes color to match the earth; the earth doesn't change color to match the chameleon." Translating genomic data of relevance to health care and response to EPID within the context of Africa cannot be done in isolation of "African cultural diversity." Culture and modern developments (such as genomics) can come together with the meeting of mutual respect, but there are social and economic challenges that need to be addressed.

Social challenges. Human genomics provides a historical record of relatedness between peoples and cultures. It is a code of our evolutionary past, human migrations, and adaptations. Genomics therefore has the potential to place people into groups or "races" leading to unity or creating (or fueling) conflict. In a continent like Africa, which has a complex cultural substructure, the impact of discovering that one's ancestral heritage may not be "as you thought" (e.g., learning your father is not your father) has the potential for significant psychological and societal impacts.

Another challenge is to avoid the use of genomic data (and infectious disease data) for cultural discrimination. Data that may suggest that one group of people is more susceptible (or likely carriers) of a disease than another has the potential for generating group-based stigmatization. There are many examples of this throughout human history. Stigmatization associated with HIV/AIDS resulted in its definition as a "homosexual disease" in the United States and as a "women's disease" in parts of Africa. Stigma associated with being HIV-positive in Africa fueled the spread of the epidemic.

Genomic data provide the tools to link specific cultural practices that may be taboo in another society to the spread of diseases. Polygamy and consanguineous marriage, for example, although fairly common throughout Africa, are frowned upon in most western cultures. If genomic data were to highlight such cultural differences, would African societies once again feel the pain of colonial-based judgment? Epidemiological data have associated specific cultural practices with the spread of infectious diseases in Africa. For example, the spread of HIV is more limited among circumcised men than their uncircumcised counterparts; gender-based inequality has been shown to increase HIV infection rates.

Because 70% of Africa's population lives in rural areas, it is important to note that the day-to-day needs will be vastly different from those in a predominantly urban western society. Public dissemination of data relevant for preventing or controlling EPID in the rural context will likely not be addressed through the standard methods of communication and technologies used in western urban societies. Rural societies are spread over vast distances, making communication and access to health care and relevant information a daily challenge, even for local governments.

Economic challenges. Cultural identity is often associated with economic status. In countries with minimal resources, the distribution of information is a significant challenge. Even if the information is available, the basic needs for survival may be overriding. Sex workers in Africa (via conversations with approximately 30 women) spoke of how the basic need for sustenance, or lack of purpose in life, were greater behavioral drivers than the fear of knowing they carried the invisible "killer germ." Economically challenged persons are not simple-minded; they are simply people without opportunities. Addressing poor economic systems will enable changes in population behavior.

Policy issues

There are specific obligations to be fulfilled in order to meet these challenges. Genomics plays a critical role (together with environment, social, and economic factors) in the creation of the global disparities in EPID. In 2010, the first African Genome Project provided a glimpse into the extent of un-captured genetic diversity. The obligation to bring genomics to Africa is summed up in the words of Archbishop Desmond Tutu: "Southern Africans are victims of many devastating diseases whose eradication requires immediate attention and international resources. My hope is that my genetic code may provide a voice for the region and serve as the starting point for a map of DNA variation significant for Southern African peoples, to be used for medical research efforts and effective design of medicines. I implore the scientific community to continue what I hope was just a first step to further medical research within the region (Tutu, 2011)." It is of global relevance that we reach out to the African community (Hayes, 2011).

Addressing the actionable next steps

- As the center of global human diversity, it is essential that Africa be included in current DNA databases that map human genome and microbiome diversity. These databases will allow for rapid prediction of EPID transmission and infection rates.

- The most critical challenge will be the prevention of discrimination-based surveillance and genomic data of relevance to EPID within extreme diverse cultural systems.

- Although global standardization is essential, one must allow for flexibility. The lessons learned during the HIV epidemic in Africa taught us that understanding and controlling the disease could not solely be based on developments happening outside Africa. Disease staging measures, gender, prevalence and mortality rates, sources of exposure, and ultimately, the genomic profile of the infecting pathogen and the infected host, differed dramatically. Information sharing needs to make room for region-specific guidelines.

- Sharing of data should also look outside the framework of the "health care professional." In many African societies, the "traditional healer" is still the primary health caregiver.

- On-the-ground education programs need to be established and run by local organizations to effectively introduce technological concepts (such as genomics) to the public. The context needs to be tangible, regionally relevant, and embrace established social structures that can reach the most rural communities.

- For the western world to be successful in Africa, it needs to raise its profile in the region and overcome historical mistrust. Economic imbalance between African and non-African communities can best be met by forming networks (bridges) among impoverished and wealthy research institutes, governments, policy makers, and scientists.

References

Hayes, V. (2011). Indigenous genomics. *Science, 332*(6030), 639.

Karenga, M. (2009, April 16). Art, struggle and African Renaissance: Fesman III. *Los Angeles Sentinel*, p. A7.

Tutu, D. (2011). Genome-sequencing anniversary: My genome. *Science, 331*(6018), 689.

** A policy position paper prepared for presentation at the conference on Emerging and Persistent Infectious Diseases (EPID): Focus on the Societal and Economic Context, convened by the Institute on Science for Global Policy (ISGP) July 8–11, 2012, at George Mason University, Fairfax, Virginia.

Debate Summary

The following summary is based on notes recorded by the ISGP staff during the not-for-attribution debate of the policy position paper prepared by Dr. Vanessa Hayes (see above). Dr. Hayes initiated the debate with a 5-minute statement of her views and then actively engaged the conference participants, including other authors, throughout the remainder of the 90-minute period. This Debate Summary represents the ISGP's best effort to accurately capture the comments offered and questions posed by all participants, as well as those responses made

by Dr. Hayes. Given the not-for-attribution format of the debate, the views comprising this summary do not necessarily represent the views of Dr. Hayes, as evidenced by her policy position paper. Rather, it is, and should be read as, an overview of the areas of agreement and disagreement that emerged from all those participating in the critical debate.

Debate conclusions

- Improved understanding of genetic variation can provide critical insights into the underlying mechanisms of infectious diseases in humans (e.g., susceptibility to a disease and progression of a disease) and lead to long-term gains in the development of therapeutics (e.g., drugs and vaccines).

- Despite the potential of genomics to aid in the prevention and control of infectious diseases, its practical applications are limited by the present data collection emphasis on individuals of European descent. To optimize its usefulness, any reference baseline for research into and applications of the human genome must accurately reflect the global diversity of genomic information from individuals from less affluent geographical regions (e.g., Africa).

- Genomic research on populations that are genetically and physically isolated from modern societies (e.g., the Bushmen in South Africa) may reveal linkages among genotype, phenotype, and the environment. Data must be collected on such isolated groups before such genetically distinct information is lost through their integration into neighboring populations.

- Stronger collaborations between regions (e.g., less-affluent and more-affluent countries) and disciplines (e.g., microbiologists and social scientists) are needed to improve the efficacy of infectious disease control programs. Ensuring that activities initiated by donor agencies are adequately maintained is also critical.

- The cultural context of a population must be considered when infectious disease control programs are implemented. Bottom-up approaches encouraging local participation in establishing prioritized strategies therefore need to be encouraged in tandem with top-down national or regional initiatives.

Current realities

Genomics, the scientific discipline that focuses on the hereditary information of an organism (encoded in either DNA or RNA) has significantly advanced during the past two decades. The progression of scientific achievements — ranging from the sequencing of the first bacterial genome in 1995 (i.e., the *Haemophilus influenzae* genome) to the completion of the Human Genome Project in 2003 — illustrates the scope and rapid pace within which the field has developed. Although scientific understanding of genomics has considerably improved, the prediction of phenotype (i.e., observable characteristics of an individual) from genotype has remained difficult to decipher due to both the influence of changing environments and the substantial number of genes that contribute to most phenotypes.

Genomics has demonstrated that humans, regardless of their geographic origin, are genetically 99% identical to one another. It was noted that the 1% difference in the genetic makeup (i.e., DNA) of humans leads not only to different appearances, but also to disparate health statuses across individuals.

Research has shown that all humans coexist with microbes (both good and bad) in and on their bodies, and that the number of microbial genes within each person exceeds the number of human genes by more than tenfold. Genomics has become a useful tool for identifying these microbes without the need for laboratory culture of organisms.

In recent years, restrictions have been placed on the sharing of biological samples outside of some countries. Such policies have generally been instituted because of intellectual property concerns that center on the fair and equitable sharing of benefits that may be derived from the biological resources within a given country. South Africa was used to illustrate restrictions. Within South Africa, trepidation related to potential outside intellectual or economic gains, which may not be reflected within the country, has led to severe limitations on the sharing of plant and animal samples and has triggered discussions on similarly limiting the distribution of human DNA samples in the future.

Societal and/or economic opportunities and challenges

Africa was a focal point of the discussion, particularly with respect to the challenges in reducing the infectious disease burden in less-affluent regions. It was noted that Africa has experienced a unique set of sociodemographic conditions that complicate efforts to control disease within the continent's borders. Africa is comprised of 54 countries, as well as more than 2,000 languages and cultures. This diversity was seen as a barrier to "one-size-fits-all" intervention approaches that do not take into account the sociocultural distinctions between and within various

African subpopulations. Additionally, the predominantly rural nature of the continent, combined with infrastructure deficiencies (e.g., roads and electrical power), were cited as impediments to ensuring that infectious disease control activities reach those who need them.

Because poverty is widespread throughout Africa, both at country and individual levels, and because sufficient resources from within these societies have not been available, contributions from donors outside Africa have provided substantial aid for infectious disease control. While many donor initiatives have been instrumental in building capacity (e.g., for molecular diagnostics), it was asserted that donors frequently shift their attention and funds (e.g., to different regions or diseases), which impedes the maintenance and long-term success of the programs they begin.

Some of the infrastructural shortfalls that have previously limited genomics research in Africa were believed to be surmountable through global technological advances. For example, it was noted that when good computational networks are instituted, scientists in Africa can work together with researchers in more-affluent countries through cloud computing. Such technology-induced cooperation means that many of the machines and staff that would otherwise physically be necessary in Africa frequently are not required. While it was suggested that the technology revolution should be capitalized on where possible, it was also cautioned that viewing new technologies as a wholesale substitute for other forms of capacity building within Africa would neglect problems that technology cannot currently address.

It was noted that even if genomics provides answers to disease susceptibility and transmission, those most in need of the drugs and vaccines created with the aid of genomic data may not experience the majority of the benefits. Research and development for such therapeutics has traditionally been expensive and therefore, the end cost of drugs and/or vaccines may be prohibitive to both individuals in less-affluent regions and impoverished individuals within more-affluent regions.

Balancing the short-term versus long-term needs of individuals throughout the world, and particularly those in Africa, was considered a significant challenge given the limited resources available globally. It was questioned whether public health measures such as the provision of fresh drinking water, vector control, immunizations, and improved nutrition — all of which impart immediate benefits on the ground — should be prioritized ahead of the longer-term gains that may be achieved through genomics research.

Avoiding discrimination based on genomic data was considered a significant challenge. While not collecting or analyzing genomic information was cited as the only way presently to guarantee that data-driven discrimination does not occur, it was also noted that this is not a realistic option. Alternatives methods for preventing data-based discrimination were believed to be needed.

Policy issues

Within the development of genomic databases, there has been a strong bias toward obtaining information from individuals of European descent. It was contended that improved understanding of global variations in human DNA sequences may lead to valuable discoveries related to human infectious disease susceptibility, and that African genomes are of particular interest because of the substantial diversity in their DNA compared with other populations. It was argued that research specifically on the genomes of the indigenous Southern African Bushmen is of critical importance. While the value in investigating an isolated population such as the Bushmen was questioned, given that most people in contemporary societies are genetically admixed (i.e., they possess new genetic lineages resulting from individuals from two or more previously separated populations interbreeding), it was argued that the Bushmen's genomes may hold clues to disentangling the linkages among genotype, phenotype, and the environment. Their genetic and physical isolation from the modern world was considered a key, distinguishing factor in this type of research. Additionally, it was emphasized that the window of opportunity to create a reference baseline using genomic data from the Bushmen may soon close because of potential population declines as well as increased mixing with surrounding populations.

HIV/AIDS, tuberculosis, and malaria, also known as "the big three" because of the substantial morbidity and mortality they cause worldwide, have reduced the life expectancy in some parts of sub-Saharan Africa to approximately half that found in more-affluent regions. While it was considered unlikely that genomics will negate the substantial health challenges caused by these and other diseases in the short term, it was contended that genomics is a critical tool for the development of long-term solutions, such as vaccines. Research has shown that improved understanding of genetic variation in humans (e.g., susceptibility to a disease and its progression) holds promise for developing therapeutic interventions. For diseases like HIV/AIDS, it was considered critical for African genetic variation to be more fully represented in research, largely due to the high prevalence of the disease on the continent, which may hold clues for the discovery of significant genetic variants. Additionally, it was noted that current research must more broadly encompass strains of diseases like HIV that mainly occur in less-affluent regions (e.g., HIV-2) for efforts to prevent and control HIV (and other diseases) to be globally effective.

The need for stronger collaborations and partnerships between regions (e.g., less-wealthy and more-wealthy countries) and disciplines was considered essential for the success of infectious disease control efforts. Such partnerships and collaborations were believed to reduce costs and increase effectiveness. For example, it was noted that scientists can answer questions that are of significance to their own countries without setting up the requisite technologies within their borders by working in tandem with researchers in other locations (e.g., through the development of strong research networks). However, it was also argued that the sustainability of partnerships must be considered so that initiatives do not launch and then founder, which has been a recurrent problem. Where donor agencies contribute to collaborations, it was recommended that a substantial portion of the overall funds be used to help maintain the programs they create.

In addition to ensuring that donors plan for the longevity of their projects, it was noted that the sustainability of infectious disease and other health improvement programs is improved when bottom-up approaches are instituted in cooperation with top-down national or regional initiatives. Engaging local representatives to participate in the decision-making processes that establish priorities and strategies was considered an important way to encourage local responsibility for implementing policies while simultaneously targeting resources to where they are most needed.

It was argued that rigid policies directed toward people from dissimilar socioeconomic backgrounds and geographies may not be as effective as flexible policies that can adapt to diverse cultures and changing environments (e.g., governmental shifts and new information). It was emphasized that although resources and/or political will for tailoring decisions to specific subpopulations may be limited, efforts need to be made to actively include the changing needs of local groups into decision-making as much as possible.

It was cautioned that lessons from past failures between the scientific community and disadvantaged populations (e.g., the Tuskegee syphilis experiment) must be carefully considered before genomic research is conducted in less-affluent countries. To mitigate damage that could be caused by a repetition of the ethical mishaps of the past, it was suggested that social scientists, natural scientists, and historians internationally work together across multiple communities to develop acceptable codes of behavior for genomics research.

Although policy makers typically give precedence to issues that presently impact their own constituencies, it was argued that this mindset is not effective for infectious disease control because globalization has accelerated the pace within which infectious diseases in one region can become problems across the world. While many countries currently address infectious disease challenges outside their borders for precisely this reason, it was noted that the emphasis of such initiatives typically centers on crises and short-term gains. Thus, building long-term investments in research, capacity-building, and other disease control activities — in parallel with short-term initiatives — were believed to be essential priorities.

While the importance of interdisciplinary research has increasingly been recognized in recent years, social and life sciences frequently still function in isolation of one another. It was argued that projects focusing on the prevention and mitigation of infectious diseases need to expand the breadth and scope of interdisciplinary cooperation. For example, it was noted that the value of genomics research for human health will substantially improve if human biology knowledge is integrated with information on the environments within which humans live (e.g., social, cultural, economic, political, and physical environments).

Communication Challenges in Managing Social and Economic Impacts of Emerging and Infectious Diseases**

Paul Slovic, Ph.D.
President, Decision Research
Professor of Psychology, University of Oregon,
Eugene, Oregon

Summary

Risk is inherently hard to understand and communicate. Analytic feeling and "gut reaction" coexist in the mind. The latter gives rise to "risk as feeling," characterized by fast, intuitive reactions, dominated by affect and emotion, and creates a fertile climate for powerful influences from culture, ideology, framing, and many cognitive and emotional biases. Risk feelings include stigmatization that may lead to avoidance of people, places, and products perceived to be abnormally risky. Effective communication is essential to reduce the direct health effects from emerging and persistent infectious diseases (EPID) and the indirect social and economic costs due to stigma, which could be enormous. Communicators need to understand the psychology of risk and conduct research to determine whether their messages are being understood and acted upon appropriately. Communication strategies must be tailored to fit the characteristics of the exposed population and the nature of the threat. Efforts to improve communication are essential and likely to be highly cost effective.

Current realities

Diverse factors, including accelerated global transport, climate change, migration, population growth, urbanization, and bioterrorism facilitate the emergence and/or spread of infectious diseases. The threat of EPID is exacerbated by problems of communication, risk perception, and decision-making.

Communication technologies are a two-edged sword. Information blankets the globe with unprecedented speed, bringing greater potential to educate, warn, and guide protective actions. At the same time, misinformation can spread quickly and uncontrollably. Print media, radio, and television are losing ground to social media, which has the potential to blur the visibility and salience of expertise and give voice to uninformed or malicious messages.

Risk, by its very nature, is hard to understand — for experts as well as laypersons. Analytic thinking and "gut reaction" coexist in the mind. The latter gives rise to "risk as feeling," characterized by fast, intuitive reactions, dominated by affect and emotion, and creates a fertile climate for powerful impacts driven by culture, ideology, framing, and cognitive and emotional biases. Intuitive thinking underestimates the importance of events large in scope described only by statistics. Stories of individual victims carry much more emotional meaning and impact, but this can lead to overreaction. Feelings underlie stigmatization of people, places, and products deemed abnormally risky. Avoidance of those stigmatized people, places, and products can lead to massive social and economic impacts, as happened during the plague in the Middle Ages and more recently with outbreaks of severe acute respiratory syndrome (SARS), H1N1 influenza, and bovine spongiform encephalopathy (BSE). These latter episodes have led to billions of dollars in losses globally.

Trust, too, is essentially a feeling state that is closely allied with perception and acceptance of risk. Trust is hard-earned, but can be permanently destroyed in an instant. As one example of the subtle biasing effect of risk as feeling, consider a rare, harmful event that is expected to occur with extremely low probability (e.g., $p = .01$). If this is communicated as occurring in 1% of exposed individuals, it will be judged much less risky than if it is communicated as occurring in 1 out of every 100 exposed persons. The latter frame stimulates thoughts and images of "the one victim," resulting in stronger negative feelings and greater perceived risk. Greater precautions will be taken as well, when the risk is described by a relative frequency (i.e., 1 out of 100). Word selection, too, is critically important. "Pandemic" creates a scarier impression than does "epidemic."

Another emotional bias is "probability neglect," occurring in people and governments facing an uncertain event that is dreadful to contemplate. For example, the strong feelings triggered by "worst-case scenarios" can lead to overreaction because people fail to take probabilities, which may be miniscule, into account. This may ultimately result in poor decision-making.

Social and/or economic opportunities and challenges

Risk communicators need to understand the subtlety and power of images and feelings, a skill that advertisers and consumer marketers have honed for decades. The Actionable Next Step emerging from the ISGP conferences concerning the development of clear, evidence-based messages for the public presents great opportunities to reduce the social and economic costs of EPID, which can be massive. Consider, for example, a bioterrorism incident, such as distribution of anthrax spores in a major urban area. Methods for studying the social and economic impacts of such events have been developed by researchers who have created a "scenario simulation" that uses video simulation of an unfolding series of local news reports to immerse respondents in the developing details of an anthrax attack in their city. Questions are designed to determine: (i) whether residents will remain in the city; (ii) what personal financial, social, and political considerations influence those decisions; (iii) what changes in perceptions and actions occur during the cleanup and recovery period; and (iv) what economic incentives can facilitate recovery. Simulation affords opportunities to intervene with various forms of education and messages to determine which lead to the most appropriate behavioral responses. For example, risk perception research suggests that giving people an understanding of what officials are doing to control and minimize exposure and harm, and what they personally can do to control the risk, is essential to mitigating the harmful consequences of actions driven by fear.

Scenarios educating people about EPID and building trust in what authorities and individuals can do to control the risk, can be thought of as a communications analogy to the biological principle of "inoculation," where a person is exposed to a mild dose of a virus to stimulate her defenses against a subsequent, stronger attack. Inoculation theory originated as a method of making people resistant to attacks on their "attitudes" and it is now gaining prominence in health campaigns and other domains. Of course, the cost of developing and testing such scenarios may be prohibitive.

Policy issues

The Area of Consensus and Actionable Next Steps in the realm of risk communication emerging from the conferences convened by the Institute on Science for Global Policy (ISGP) are broad in scope, and therefore, it is difficult to identify major flaws in them. Yet, it would be helpful for there to be more specificity in these recommendations. To augment the current Actionable Next Steps, several recommendations can be made. The cognitive and behavioral issues raised here fall within the broader recommendations provided in a previous policy position paper by Viswanath (2012), which include: (i) the development of a transnational risk information and communication architecture; (ii) investment in human capital to assess, interpret, and communicate risks of EPID expeditiously; (iii) investment in the science, dissemination, and implementation of evidence-based risk communication strategies; and (iv) promotion of access to information to mitigate inequalities in exposure to beneficial messages.

Within this broad evidence-based framework, additional guidelines can be proposed:

- Conduct empirical research, including scenario simulation studies, to determine whether messages are understood and acted upon appropriately. Good risk messages are inherently difficult to create and cannot be trusted without some degree of testing. The good news is that communication can be studied rather easily — much can be learned by simply asking people or focus groups to read and react to proposed messages. Much more sophisticated methods, such as scenario simulation, can also be employed effectively if time and resources permit.

- Scientific organizations such as the International Union of Toxicology have sponsored risk assessment short courses to educate young scientists from around the world. Similar international courses should be developed and offered to train communicators. The payoff in reduced mortality and reduced social and economic disruption resulting from EPID could be enormous.

- Communicators need to appreciate that risk messages are politically sensitive. Frightening messages can stigmatize a region, resulting in economic losses even if the disease threat does not materialize. When a threat is uncertain, officials may stifle communication to prevent stigmatization.

- Clearly there can be no "one size fits all" model for communication. Strategies must be culturally appropriate and sensitive to diversity of population backgrounds, resources, and available technologies as well as being tailored to the diverse nature of threats from EPID.

References

Compton, J. A., & Pfau, M. (2005). Inoculation theory of resistance to influence at maturity: Recent progress in theory development and application and suggestions for future research. *Communication Yearbook, 29*, 97–145.

John, R. (2012). *A dynamic portrayal of public decision making during recovery from a biological terrorist attack on a major U.S. city*. Los Angeles, CA: National Center for Risk and Economic Analysis of Terrorism Events, University of Southern California.

Viswanath, K. (2012). *Communicating risk in an age of information plenty: Implications for policy and practice of Emerging and Persistent Infectious Diseases (EPID)*. In Institute on Science for Global Policy (Eds.), *Emerging and Persistent Infectious Diseases: Focus on Mitigation* (pp. 41–45). Tucson, AZ: ISGP.

*** A policy position paper prepared for presentation at the conference on Emerging and Persistent Infectious Diseases (EPID): Focus on the Societal and Economic Context, convened by the Institute on Science for Global Policy (ISGP) July 8–11, 2012, at George Mason University, Fairfax, Virginia.*

Debate Summary

The following summary is based on notes recorded by the ISGP staff during the not-for-attribution debate of the policy position paper prepared by Dr. Paul Slovic (see above). Dr. Slovic initiated the debate with a 5-minute statement of his views and then actively engaged the conference participants, including other authors, throughout the remainder of the 90-minute period. This Debate Summary represents the ISGP's best effort to accurately capture the comments offered and questions posed by all participants, as well as those responses made by Dr. Slovic. Given the not-for-attribution format of the debate, the views comprising this summary do not necessarily represent the views of Dr. Slovic, as evidenced by his policy position paper. Rather, it is, and should be read as, an overview of the areas of agreement and disagreement that emerged from all those participating in the critical debate.

Debate conclusions

- Developing effective risk communication requires a clear and accurate understanding of the cultural perceptions of risk within each society, as well as of the specific worldview and values that shape such perceptions. Although compared with other interventions, such as drug development for infectious diseases, timely risk communication is low-cost and simple. Its effectiveness often depends on engaging local individuals who understand the specific cultural mores and who can serve as the liaison between the messenger and the message recipients.

- Risk communication is complicated by people's limited understanding of the meaning of data, probability, and uncertainty. Convincing people to move beyond their emotional assessment of risk and to think analytically is a challenge for essentially all risk communicators.

- To maximize effectiveness of risk communication, messages should be: (i) packaged in the form of stories, narratives, and anecdotes, (ii) varied depending on the stage of an event (i.e., people want to know something different immediately after an event than later), (iii) conveyed through trusted messengers, and (iv) crafted in advance after some testing with risk communicators and scientists. Risk communicators also need to appropriately time their messages to avoid delivering information too early (which may unnecessarily instill fear) or too late (which may be unhelpful or promote distrust).

- The recent increase in information on risk from the Internet and social media has changed the way risk messages are received and acted upon by the public. The impact of communication from authorities has declined because the public cannot necessarily assess a messenger's level of knowledge, expertise, or influence. The public health community needs to be actively engaged in social media to counter the influence of false and misleading messages.

- Educational efforts are needed to improve the ability of the general population, including children, to properly assess risks via rational analysis (i.e., deliberate, analytical thinking) and to avoid decisions based primarily on emotional responses.

Current realities

Since a standard definition of "risk" has not been widely established or accepted, the effective communication of risk to both the public and decision makers remains complicated and often difficult to achieve. Definitions of risk vary depending on the professional context within which they are developed (e.g., actuaries versus medical professions). They include different meanings such as: (i) risk as a hazard (e.g., a potentially risky event or occurrence, such as a nuclear accident), (ii) risk as a probability (e.g., the chance of something occurring), and (iii) risk as a consequence (e.g., the possibility of getting a ticket for allowing a parking meter to expire).

Humans simultaneously process information about risks in two contradictory ways: affect or feelings (i.e., the fast, intuitive gut reaction) and reason or analysis (i.e., the slow, thoughtful, scientific way of analyzing risk). In the ancient world, risk assessments were primarily based on gut feelings and experience (e.g., by processing questions such as, "How does the water smell?" or "Did I get sick when I drank the water?"). In the modern world, science (e.g., analytic chemistry, toxicology) can be used to measure and identify even very small risks. The addition of this scientific information frequently complicates the ability of the human mind to determine a hazard's level of risk because such information often conflicts with an individual's gut instincts.

On an evolutionary timescale, humans have only recently become capable of and interested in thinking more abstractly about risk (e.g., worrying about things that cannot be seen or events that are happening in other parts of the world). It was noted that people generally make decisions about risks based on feelings that stem from past experiences instead of conducting explicit risk calculations. It was contended that in many situations (e.g., deciding when it is safe to change lanes while driving or whether it is safe to walk down a dark street) feelings are valid and beneficial for split-second decision-making. Under other circumstances, feelings do not always produce appropriate reactions because they can be misleading (particularly when an experience is new or when messages are crafted in ways that over- or under-stimulate certain emotions).

Risk communication necessitates an understanding of people's perceptions of risk. Risk perceptions are greatly influenced by the unique set of factors that comprise a risk or hazard (e.g., whether the exposure is voluntary or involuntary, controllable or uncontrollable, or leads to immediate versus delayed consequences). The values held by individuals that relate to these factors play an important role in how risk is perceived and accepted. For example, exposure to radiation from sources of nuclear energy is generally perceived as having a high level of risk because it is often viewed as relatively uncontrolled, involuntary, and capable of causing severe consequences. By contrast, medical uses of radiation (e.g., medical X-rays) have been more widely accepted. It was also noted that people commonly view situations or actions as either risky or safe with little middle ground between the two ends of the spectrum.

Some societies (e.g., parts of the world with lower life expectancies) were considered more heavily exposed to risk than other populations. Questions were raised regarding what level of risk is acceptable, as well as whether people who live in such societies are less sensitive to risk because they have built up a tolerance to potential hazards.

Most people have not been educated about concepts related to risk or probability. While science relies heavily on probability, many in the public are not educated about how to think probabilistically since formal courses on risk and probability generally are not taught to many students in high school or college. Education on risk and probability typically is only provided to the small percentage of the global population who take statistics courses in college or graduate school. It was argued that probability is as important as other mathematical sciences, but is a neglected course of study by the educational system.

Social and/or economic opportunities and challenges

The effective communication of risk to the public and to policy makers is frequently complicated by the difficulties many have in considering issues analytically. People often assess issues of risk emotionally rather than methodically considering the accepted facts.

There routinely have been significant differences between evidence-based risk calculations determined by scientists and the evaluation of risk based on emotions where perceptions of risk are greatly influenced by cultural factors and societal values. For effective risk messaging to be formulated, there is a need for cultural and societal issues to be understood and not dismissed as irrelevant (e.g., when they do not align with technical assessments of a risk). To obtain an understanding of such specific worldviews, the messaging concerning risk needs to be shaped in cooperation with those who understand the specific society and who can act as a liaison to the recipients of the messages.

The efforts to properly communicate risk were also considered to be complicated by limitations in the public's understanding of data and uncertainty. The public tends to use different rules and heuristics than statisticians to decipher scientific findings. For example, statisticians understand that the accuracy of findings improves with larger sample sizes while lay individuals often believe that one can be as confident in the statistics derived from a small sample of data as in a large one.

It was also noted that the wide availability of social media has significantly changed the way risk messages are received and acted upon by the public. The recent increase in information communicated via the Internet and social media (e.g., Twitter) was considered a significant barrier to effective risk communication. The control of authoritative information by officials has been "lost." Although people often use the Internet as their primary source of information, they generally cannot assess the level of knowledge or authority of the messenger. Messages conveyed over social media are often conveyed in the form of stories or narratives which are especially powerful in influencing public opinion through emotional responses.

Because of the complex, subtle way that the mind is thought to react to information about risk, it was argued that it is difficult to predict how to optimize a message concerning risk without conducting risk communication research before creating a message. Risk communication has been viewed as relatively easy to study and costs less than other interventions associated with risk mitigation (e.g., drug development for diseases). By determining how people perceive hazards, culturally sensitive messages can be formulated to minimize misinterpretations of risks.

Misunderstandings of risk have the capacity to cause overreactions. When individuals assess risk through rational analysis, various dimensions of risk are taken into account, including the severity of consequences and the likelihood of the event. However, when risks with potentially severe outcomes (e.g., terrorist actions) are evaluated via feelings, individuals frequently overlook the true probability of an occurrence and act as though the threat is more likely than in reality. Evaluating risks without properly analyzing the probability of an event can lead to inappropriately allocating financial and human resources.

In some cases, the incorrect perception of risk leads to underreactions. People often maintain cognitive bias against what is considered "normal" for a society (e.g., persistent, as opposed to novel, infectious diseases) even when such threats may be dangerous. Underreactions to risks can be just as problematic as overreactions. For example, an inherent bias against persistent diseases has limited funding for endemic disease control relative to the resources allocated to address threats from novel diseases.

The challenge found in measuring and conveying the risk associated with different types of situations (e.g., chemical terrorism versus endemic diseases) has been of major concern and has been complicated by the absence of a common language to describe risk. For example, the difficulties that government agencies experienced when working together to set the color-coded terrorism threat alert levels illustrated the problems associated with the subjectivity of risk measurement. While recognizing that agreeing on a specific set of parameters and variables is challenging, it was proposed that there is significant value in developing a common algorithm or scoring system for assessing the risk of different events (e.g., infectious diseases, terrorist).

Concern was expressed that there is only a small, fragmented community of risk communicators. Since most research on the psychology of risk assessment has been conducted within western populations, there is also a deficiency in our understanding of how other cultures think about risk.

The relationship between authorities and their constituencies is a critical issue that has been challenging to resolve. It is important that policy makers are prepared to respond to their constituents' concerns related to risk assessment regardless of whether these concerns are well-founded and based on actual risks. Government priorities and responses related to potential risks are often influenced by advocacy efforts, as well as by how the public perceives and responds emotionally to risks. Passion was said to often be more influential than data and evidence. Such decisions can lead to a disproportionate allocation of resources and attention in response to issues that pose minimal health risks.

Policy issues

It was recognized that political considerations can be directly associated with the assessment of risks and the related messages to the public. Because there are so many ways to define and measure risk, risk assessments may be "tweake[d] and torture[d]" so they legitimize the actions of a specific group and/or reflect a particular viewpoint. Officials may sometimes stifle communication when a threat is uncertain to prevent the stigmatization of people or places and/or to minimize activities that can negatively impact an economy or region.

When conveying information about risk, policy makers need to frame messages as stories, narratives, and anecdotes. Policy makers also need to have an accurate understanding of the credibility of the scientific research underlying the stories. Risk communication messages should vary depending on the stage of an event because what the public immediately wants to know frequently differs from the information they require at a later point in time. The timing within which risk information is communicated was also viewed as important because there is a balance between communicating about risks too early (which may be unwarranted and spread fear) and communication that comes too late (which may be unhelpful or promote distrust in authorities). Providing overly-charged information was discouraged because sensationalized messages may create an "air raid mentality" that leads to undesirable outcomes such as unwarranted economic losses and social unrest.

Conveying messages through trusted messengers was noted as an especially important component of effective risk communication. To ensure maximum effectiveness of risk messaging, the risk communication community must work with scientists and well-known public figures to ensure the credibility of each message. Testing these messages among a large community of experts in advance of their dissemination can also ensure their impact. Cooperating with well-known public figures who do not necessarily understand the scientific basis for the messages can also be a critical step in building public acceptance.

The importance of the context within which risk messages are framed was repeatedly highlighted. Risk comparisons (e.g., nuclear power is safer than driving a car) are useful ways to explain risks since they connect the information provided with the probability of an event occurring. While some have rejected the use of risk comparisons due to instances where comparisons have been unsuccessful (primarily due to communicators who were viewed as being manipulative), it was argued that they are often a valuable tool.

Communication during the 2009 "swine flu" influenza pandemic (PDM 2009 H1N1) was presented as an example of successful risk messaging. The effective components of the risk communication strategy for H1N1 pandemic in the United States included that (i) messages were created in advance of the first case, (ii) messages were unified (e.g., four consistent talking points used by federal agencies),

(iii) continual updates were provided to the public (including what was known and unknown), and (iv) messaging was delivered by a source with authority. Research in Canada showed that during the H1N1 outbreak, daily public updates by national authorities, which were positive (i.e., included updates on the progress of immunization) and personable, led to increased immunization rates. The 2001 U.S. anthrax attacks were presented as an example of unsuccessful risk communication because the messages that were conveyed were not consonant with the threat.

It was urged that scientists need to play a more active role in communicating the findings of their research to help the public correctly interpret the meaning of their studies. A transnational coalition of worldwide scientists, health professionals, and policy makers is needed to develop a coordinated system to align risk communication across countries and issues. As social media become an increasingly important source of information, the public health community needs to learn how to effectively utilize it in its various forms to counter false messages (e.g., that vaccines cause autism).

While requiring time and expertise, scenario-based testing was agreed to be a practical and useful approach for evaluating risk communication messages in advance of an event. By building a time frame into a scenario (e.g., a dirty bomb explosion that is cleaned up in 30 days), stage-specific reactions to a particular risk can be more effectively gauged and subsequently integrated into messages to the public. Scenario studies can also help to assess the potential direct and indirect consequences and costs of an event, including direct damages (e.g., fatalities, injuries, and property damage) and "ripple effects" of behavior that may impact economic costs to a region.

It was suggested that educational efforts to help the public properly evaluate different risks using analyses of credible information, as opposed to primarily their emotions, is an important element in preparing any society for an emergency. Enhancing the degree to which people think analytically (i.e., carefully, slowly, and deliberately) about risks is therefore considered of significant value to officials for improving the outcome of emergency situations.

Synthetic Biology: Ethical and Social Challenges**

Arthur L. Caplan, Ph.D.
Division of Medical Ethics
New York University Langone Medical Center,
New York City, New York

Summary

The promise of synthetic biology is enormous. The technology can be used to help solve some of the greatest challenges now facing humanity including the production of more food, energy, clean water, and safer, more effective vaccines and medicines. The technology required involves the genetic modification of viruses, bacteria, and microbes and that raises numerous ethical questions. Is there adequate regulatory oversight, environmental protection, and vigilance against the misuse of the technology by amateurs or terrorists? Other concerns involve the moral acceptability of creating novel life forms. In grappling with both types of issues there is, as yet, no consensus on which principled moral stance is appropriate: precaution or prudence.

Current realities

The promise of synthetic biology is enormous. The technology can be used to help solve some of the greatest challenges now facing humanity including the production of more food, energy, arable land, and clean water, the control of pollution, and the creation of safer more effective vaccines and medicines. The technology can also be used to create biological incubators that can accelerate many biochemical production processes.

Yet, the technology involves the genetic modification of viruses, bacteria, and microbes, and this raises numerous ethical questions.

Social and ethical challenges

At present there is insufficient regulatory oversight and environmental protection governing synthetic biology. There is a risk of the misuse of the technology by amateurs or terrorists and accidents also pose an important danger. Other concerns involve the moral acceptability of drastically altering existing life forms or creating novel life forms. In grappling with these issues there is, as yet, no consensus on the principled moral stance that is appropriate: precaution or prudence.

In facing the risks associated with synthetic biology, two schools of thought have emerged: precaution and stewardship or prudence. However, there are divergent opinions regarding which is the appropriate moral stance toward emerging technologies such as synthetic biology.

The first school of thought, precaution, is predominant in Western Europe. This view maintains that the burden of coping with risk falls on those who would innovate any new technology. The "precautionary principle" holds that if an action or innovation has a risk of causing harm to the public or the environment then the burden of proof that it is not harmful falls on those who propose the action or innovation. They must demonstrate the absence of risk before a technology such as synthetic biology can be implemented.

This principle sets an extraordinarily high bar for coping with risk. It asks that risk be proven to be zero or so low as to be irrelevant with a high degree of confidence.

Some have argued that new technologies such as synthetic biology require a different moral stance, which I and others term "responsible prudence."

Based on the responsible prudence view, the proper response to risk is to determine the extent to which risk exists and then to institute a plan of action that ensures adequate oversight, accountability, liability, risk minimization, and transparency.

Some will argue that altering microbes is inherently wrong. No degree of social or economic benefit could justify the hubris of trying to design artificial life forms that can serve human purposes. "Playing God" is the form this objection almost always takes.

Oddly, no major religion has any objections based on principle to altering the natural world. Religion has long ago come to terms with medicine, forestry, agriculture, aquaculture, and mining. Religious concerns are more focused on the equity with which benefits are to be distributed and the purposes to which synthetic biology might be put.

In worrying about playing God, it is more the "playing" than the "God" part of the objection that carries moral weight. If scientists or industry are seen as unaccountable for what they do, if there is no transparency about the uses to which synthetic biology is put, if amateurs are seen as being able to muck around with nature simply for fun or curiosity, then the unease around allowing synthetic biology to advance could well be the basis for either hindering its application or even banning the technology.

Policy options

- The key risk posed by synthetic biology is the release of engineered organisms into the natural environment where they could interact with naturally occurring living entities in ways that could cause harm to ecosystems or human health. Releases could be the result of accident, incompetency, deliberate intent, or industrial release as waste or by-products.

- Those advocating the precautionary principle will find any risk sufficient to block the introduction of synthetic organisms into the environment. Prudentialists will argue for the creation of clear government oversight and duties, liability for any damage done, the branding of organisms to permit easy identification and tracking, the creation of fragile organisms so they cannot flourish outside controlled environments, and some restriction on access to information and techniques to minimize misuse by amateurs or terrorists.

- The recent battle over publishing the formula for synthesizing deadly strains of pandemic flu illustrates a policy of allowing synthetic biology to evolve, but with restrictions that can limit risk.

References

President's Commission for the Study of Bioethical Issues on Bioethics Report on Synthetic Biology: http://bioethics.gov/cms/sites/default/files/PCSBI-Synthetic-Biology-Report-12.16.10.pdf.

Caplan, A. (2012). Get a grippe: lessons learned from the controversy over publication of pandemic flu research. *Health Affairs Blog*, 8 May 2012, http://healthaffairs.org/blog/2012/05/08/get-a-grippe-lessons-learned-from-the-controversy-over-publication-of-pandemic-flu-research/.

*** A policy position paper prepared for presentation at the conference on Emerging and Persistent Infectious Diseases (EPID): Focus on the Societal and Economic Context, convened by the Institute on Science for Global Policy (ISGP) July 8–11, 2012, at George Mason University, Fairfax, Virginia.*

Debate Summary

The following summary is based on notes recorded by the ISGP staff during the not-for-attribution debate of the policy position paper prepared by Prof. Arthur Caplan (see above). Prof. Caplan initiated the debate with a 5-minute statement of his views and then actively engaged the conference participants, including other authors, throughout the remainder of the 90-minute period. This Debate Summary represents the ISGP's best effort to accurately capture the comments offered and questions posed by all participants, as well as those responses made by Prof. Caplan. Given the not-for-attribution format of the debate, the views comprising this summary do not necessarily represent the views of Prof. Caplan, as evidenced by his policy position paper. Rather, it is, and should be read as, an overview of the areas of agreement and disagreement that emerged from all those participating in the critical debate.

Debate conclusions

- There are serious, ongoing debates concerning how to optimize the benefits anticipated from the development of synthetic biology while protecting the public from any potential disadvantages arising from its applications. Three overarching frameworks, based on the distinct principles of precaution, stewardship, and reasonable prudence, have been proposed. Each framework appeals to different types of stakeholders. While more extensive discussions are required to reach a consensus, reasonable prudence and, to a lesser degree, stewardship both garnered significant support.

- Alleviating public concerns regarding the potential risks associated with synthetic biology was considered critical if its benefits are to be realized. Although the synthetic biology community has tried to ease public anxiety through efforts to self-regulate, it remains to be determined whether these efforts have been sufficiently effective. While instituting clear oversight, accountability, and transparency are potentially valuable steps toward gaining the public's trust, concerns remain that dominating governmental control will stifle innovation.

- Liability measures, such as monetary fines, criminal penalties, and/or research suspensions, may be beneficial tools for ensuring that the synthetic biology community is responsible for potential adverse events. However, identifying and enforcing penalties that are appropriate to any transgressions is challenging, especially since liability measures that threaten entire enterprises could limit innovative research in the field.

- It remains unclear how much formal regulation, as opposed to best practices and guidelines, is required to prevent and mitigate accidental or intentional synthetic biology hazards. Postponing decisions on establishing a regulatory apparatus, however, could result in reactive policies (i.e., stemming from a crisis) that are instituted without input from the synthetic biology community (e.g., by the courts).

Current realities

Debates regarding the value of synthetic biology largely have centered on divergent perceptions of the relative benefits versus risks of the resultant technology. The spectrum of opinions has spanned those who argue that the prospective benefits to society for remedying current global challenges (e.g., infectious disease control, food supplies, energy sources, and climate change) are so great that they outweigh the potential risks (e.g., protecting the environment from accidental release and misuse of designed organisms by amateurs or terrorists), to those who maintain that the potential dangers are serious enough to prevent synthetic biology from being pursued under any circumstances.

Three moral frameworks were outlined as current options for promoting responsible research and development while protecting the public from potential hazards: the precautionary principle, stewardship, and reasonable prudence.

The precautionary principle represents the view that those who wish to execute a technology must first prove that any suspected risks (e.g., to the public or environment) are completely unfounded before they can take action. It was noted that the precautionary principle is more popular in Europe than in other regions of the world.

The stewardship approach, as opposed to the precautionary principle, is based on conducting ongoing and coordinated reviews of the field's risks but intervening only if problems materialize. Proponents of such "watchful waiting" argue that it serves to both promote innovation and protect the public. Stewardship has been the dominant framework in the United States and is supported by the U.S. Presidential Commission for the Study of Bioethical Issues.

Reasonable prudence represents a third approach by advocating efforts to err on the side of risk to promote innovation in concert with adequate oversight, accountability, and transparency.

Although those who support the precautionary principle support blocking the research and applications of synthetic biology until all risks can be removed, banning the development of this technology was not considered a viable option since there is currently no clear distinction between "synthetic" and "other" forms of biology.

"Don't play God," a line of reasoning against synthetic biology technologies, was considered a purely secular argument, as opposed to a theological contention. It was asserted that religious traditions generally do not have any principle-based objections to the manipulation of nature and that the primary issue underlying the "don't play God" argument is a fear that scientists will not be held accountable for their actions.

The synthetic biology community has actively tried to address biosafety and biosecurity concerns by promoting self-regulation, ethics and safety training, and internal committee reviews. Yet it was noted that, in reality, the field has not been completely self-governed. Synthetic biology research conducted with federal money has been subject to reviews by funding bodies. Additionally, synthetic biologists have been required to follow rigorous procedures when attempting to patent an invention.

Public concern regarding the potential risks associated with the practice of synthetic biology has garnered increased consideration by some federal governments. This was exemplified by the U.S. Presidential Commission for the Study of Bioethical Issues, which was recently asked to respond to such concerns by identifying ways to maximize public benefits and minimize risks in this field. The Presidential Commission determined that there is no need to halt research or impose new regulations on synthetic biology; instead, the Presidential Commission recommended that five ethical principles be adopted for guiding evaluations of synthetic biology and related policy recommendations: public beneficence, responsible stewardship, intellectual freedom and responsibility, democratic deliberation, and justice and fairness.

It has been recognized that risk perception differs significantly across geographies and cultures. This was exemplified by a discussion on some of the disparate risk views held in Europe and the U.S. For instance, it was noted that the sale of raw milk is generally permissible in Europe, but not in the U.S. and that Europeans are more resistant to accepting hormones and antibiotics in their food than most Americans. It was contended that cultural differences, including the influence of environmental surroundings, have a greater impact than empirical scientific evidence on shaping risk perceptions.

It was recognized that the synthetic biology community is comprised of diverse stakeholders with competing interests. Five primary groups were identified as central to discussions on the future of this scientific field: academia, industry, do-it-yourselfers, nefarious groups or individuals, and governments.

Social and/or economic opportunities and challenges

Negative public perceptions of synthetic biology were considered one of the greatest potential barriers to the future successful development of technologies and applications of the field. It was argued that when the public is uncomfortable with a new technology, funding for research (especially by government agencies) may become impaired and limits may be placed on research (e.g., who can conduct investigations, what specific activities are permissible, and where research can be carried out).

Gaining consensus on which framework (i.e., precautionary principle, stewardship, or reasonable prudence) should be adopted to address synthetic biology concerns was considered a significant challenge since each option appeals to different societal audiences, each of which have competing interests and different degrees of comfort with risk.

It was proposed that applying the precautionary principle to synthetic biology would stifle innovation because it sets an exceedingly high bar of proving there is no risk before an action or policy can be implemented. Due largely to the potential benefits and relatively lower costs of synthetic biology, it was noted that it is extremely unlikely that the precautionary principle will ever be universally supported worldwide. Additionally, countries that adopt the precautionary principle were viewed as being at a competitive disadvantage compared with countries that adopt other frameworks for addressing synthetic biology concerns.

It was questioned whether stewardship (i.e., watchful waiting), the most broadly supported framework in the U.S., is a sustainable approach because it does not fully address public anxiety regarding the potential dangers of synthetic biology. Moreover, it was noted that a backlash against the stewardship approach, wherein the development of innovative technologies is hindered by significantly stricter controls, is a realistic possibility should an accidentally or intentionally harmful incident take place.

Because the synthetic biology community widely promotes self-regulation, it was suggested that the government regulation and oversight components of reasonable prudence would be barriers to scientists' acceptance of this framework.

Although efforts have been made to create synthetic biology best practices and codes of conduct, attention was called to the fact that these have neither been standardized nor formally implemented within or between countries. While best practices and codes of conduct are positive steps toward minimizing risk, it was noted that there are many challenges to enforcing these agreements if no process for official oversight is in place.

Enterprise-threatening liabilities were considered a substantial barrier to private industry efforts to develop the synthetic biology field fully. The issue was considered akin to liability problems that arose following the 9/11 World Trade Center attacks. Post-9/11, there was a clear need for homeland security products, but companies were unwilling to jeopardize their entire enterprises for one device, should it fail, when they could create other devices that were less risky. The U.S. accordingly created public policy in response to the need for homeland security technologies (i.e., a liability protection regime for industry under the United States Safety Act). It was suggested that the challenge of mitigating industry's liability concerns could be addressed, as was done post-9/11, by creating liability protection measures for private corporations that are coupled with accountability procedures.

Following the laboratory development of a more contagious, but not necessarily more lethal, form of H5N1 avian influenza at the University of Wisconsin-Madison and a more contagious and lethal form of H5N1 at Erasmus Medical Center, debates regarding whether such research should be censored from publication have intensified. At the center of such discussions have been concerns that lone scientists or bioterrorist groups with nefarious intentions could use published information to replicate the work. The practicality of restricting public access to synthetic biology information or techniques, however, was considered a significant challenge because research is often widely shared prior to publication. Moreover, data are frequently emailed or otherwise distributed in unencrypted formats. It was therefore believed that publication restrictions might slow the spread of confidential information, but that such an approach will not be a panacea. The issues associated with how such research data are distributed were considered in need of further debate.

Policy issues

A strong case was made for applying the reasonable prudence framework to synthetic biology public policy. It was argued that reasonable prudence may not flawlessly appease all stakeholders, but it constitutes a reasonable middle ground within the spectrum of views. It promotes technological innovation (i.e., by discouraging sweeping bans) while proactively minimizing risk (e.g., by designating responsibility to specific groups, establishing clear oversight and duties for agencies, and instituting accountability and liability for individual practitioners and/or institutions). While the reasonable prudence framework garnered significant support during the discussion, the sentiment was not unanimous. Some individuals advocated for the stewardship framework due primarily to concerns that synthetic biology is still too new a field for appropriate regulations to be identified and applied without producing negative ramifications in the future. A minority opinion in favor of the precautionary principle was also expressed by those who believed the potential risks associated with synthetic biology outweigh the potential benefits.

To minimize the potential for harm, it was suggested that liability measures should be instituted. Proposed measures included monetary fines, criminal penalties, and/or research suspensions. However, designing sufficiently rigorous penalties — particularly if substantial harm is caused by a negative incident — was considered difficult to achieve. Additionally, it was argued that liability measures must be balanced against ensuring that reasonable levels of liability protection are also afforded to researchers and industry so they can responsibly innovate without risking negative impacts on their entire enterprises.

While the transfer of synthetic biology technology from academia to industry was viewed as still being in its infancy, questions arose regarding the potential policy implications of industry's greater future involvement. The discussion primarily focused on whether the public would accept self-regulation within companies, particularly given that past examples of subpar industry self-regulation (e.g., Monsanto's dismissal of stakeholder concerns regarding genetically modified crops) have made the public increasingly wary of affording complete control to commercial enterprises.

Should an intentionally or accidentally negative incident occur, it was posited that one likely outcome would be tortuous lawsuits that ultimately increase synthetic biology regulation through the court system. It was argued that this reactive scenario is not ideal because policies that respond to disasters frequently err on the side of being overly restrictive, as well as because judicially mandated rulings are defined by nonscientists. Conversely, proactive regulations could be more limited in scope and could be informed by discussions with both synthetic biology scientists and professional societies.

Examples from other scientific fields were discussed as potential models for future synthetic biology regulation. For instance, regulations akin to those used in the nuclear weapons field (e.g., clearance restrictions, facility mandates) were suggested as a prospective way forward; however, many felt the regulatory mechanisms employed for nuclear weapons may not be directly transferable to synthetic biology. Reasons given as probable regulatory differences were that synthetic biology is a much larger field (i.e., more laboratories and practitioners than nuclear research) and that bioweapons can be created in isolated environments by a lone individual and/or small groups, whereas nuclear weapons cannot be developed in isolation. The U.S. Federal Policy for the Protection of Human Subjects was also pinpointed as a potential regulatory model because it clearly outlines areas such as oversight, review processes, and approval processes, which some individuals considered procedures that should be applied to synthetic biology.

Improving the traceability of organisms engineered through synthetic biology techniques was considered an important safety measure that can be taken. It was argued that traceability could be improved by requiring synthetic biologists to sign their work (i.e., inserting their names into a digital code within the DNA of an engineered organism). Although many synthetic biologists do adhere to this practice already, it was believed that mandating branding would ensure that negative events can be traced back to the original institution or scientists responsible, as well as signal warnings (i.e., red flags) where synthetically engineered organisms are not signed.

Those with nefarious intentions, whether lone individuals or bioterrorist groups, were considered to pose serious challenges with respect to ensuring the safety of synthetic biology. It was strongly urged that attempts be made to instill some defense mechanisms against such threats. Gathering intelligence to identify the synthetic biology activities of potentially dangerous people was considered one possible option to pursue. In addition, it was suggested that the development of protection devices to guard against biological weapons, such as specific vaccines and therapeutic procedures, should be pursued.

Which government agencies, in the U.S. and internationally, have responsibility for the oversight of synthetic biology activities or applications remains to be clarified. While the degree of regulatory power that an agency should hold was deemed subject to further discussion, it was suggested that endowing one or more agencies in a given country with an accountability role would move such conversations forward and help ease the public's safety concerns. Given the potential international impact of synthetic biology, efforts to establish some coordination among government agencies was also viewed as desirable.

How Can We Predict, Prevent and Pay
for the Next Pandemic?**

Peter Daszak, Ph.D.
President, EcoHealth Alliance, New York City, New York

Summary

The emergence of novel pandemics causes substantial mortality, morbidity, and economic loss. Recent analyses show that disease emergence is linked closely to human activity such as deforestation, agricultural intensification, and other forms of rapid economic development. Predictive models show that diseases emerge from emerging infectious disease (EID) "hotspots" in the tropics, and that they gravitate to richer countries via the global network of travel and trade. Dealing with this threat will require: (i) a "Smart Surveillance" strategy that uses predictive modeling to target hotspots for pathogen identification, together with programs that alter high-risk behaviors, and (ii) a way to levy payments to insure against pandemic emergence. This payment system will most likely need to be a form of insurance program, the cost of which would most likely be borne by the private sector or government agencies that engage in the activities that drive disease emergence in hotspot countries.

Current realities

New pandemics have emerged repeatedly in the last few decades, causing substantial mortality, morbidity, and economic loss. Most pandemics are caused by pathogens that "spill over" from their wildlife hosts (e.g., severe acute respiratory syndrome [SARS]), that evolve resistance to antibiotics (e.g., extremely drug-resistant tuberculosis [XDR TB]), that are carried to new regions with their vectors (e.g., West Nile virus), or that emerge from intensive agriculture and global food delivery networks (e.g., H1N1 and H5N1 influenzas). Even diseases that do not cause significant mortality can cause substantial economic damage through disruption of trade networks (e.g., a decline in travel to Southeast Asia during the 2002–2003 SARS outbreak) or through public response to the negative publicity surrounding a new pathogen (e.g., the decline in pork consumption during the 2009 "swine flu" influenza pandemic [PDM 2009 H1N1]) (Brahmbhatt, 2005).

Analysis of all disease emergence events for the past six decades reveals a number of predictable patterns (Jones et al., 2008): (i) disease emergence is strongly linked to human societal activity on the planet, such as land use change, intensification of agriculture, and other forms of economic development; (ii) the number of new emerging diseases is increasing annually, even after correcting for increased surveillance; and (iii) diseases with the most potential to become pandemic emerge from regions in the tropics with high biodiversity and intense human activity.

Using this information, we can map the regions on the planet most likely to propagate the next emerging disease. These EID hotspots are the major sources of new pathogens with pandemic potential. However, due to intensely interconnected patterns of global travel and trade, pathogens are able to spread rapidly and threaten lives and economies globally. In fact, emerging pandemics will rapidly gravitate to richer economies with higher levels of trade and air travel (see figure 1).

Social and/or economic opportunities and challenges

There are two unique opportunities to deal with the pandemic threat in our generation. First, the understanding of the process of disease emergence has developed rapidly so that we can predict the regions on the planet most likely to be the origin of a new disease and the populations most likely to be affected. Second, new methods for pathogen discovery make it possible to identify a substantial proportion of the unknown pathogens harbored by animal hosts before they emerge in people.

However, progress in developing a global strategy to deal with new EIDs is hampered by a lack of international capacity, even following the development of the International Health Regulations (IHR) (i.e., global rules that bind 194 countries to assist the international community in the prevention of, and response to, acute public health risks). National surveillance infrastructure in the less-wealthy countries where diseases often first emerge is usually less well funded compared to the more-wealthy countries that often bear a greater economic impact from emerging pandemics. Trade in animals and their products is poorly regulated for the spread of novel emerging pathogens, despite the World Organisation for Animal Health (OIE) regulations for known agents. Finally, there is a significant urgency to develop a global program to deal with the pandemic threat. Our analysis of the economic costs of pandemics suggests that, given a continued rise in the annual number of new diseases, there is a window of between 3 and 34 years to address the threat before it becomes too costly.

Disease emergence is therefore a classic tragedy of the commons dilemma, whereby emergence in one country (often a less-wealthy country) can have the highest impacts on another country once a pathogen enters the globalized travel and trade network. A global strategy to deal with such EIDs will be costly and there is significant uncertainty around who should pay for this and how much it will cost.

One opportunity for **predicting and identifying the next emerging zoonosis** is a "Smart Surveillance" strategy that uses predictive models to identify hotspots where zoonoses will most likely emerge. Given finite global resources for surveillance, it follows that they could be targeted to these EID hotspots to maximize the opportunity for identifying a new EID. Because zoonoses are responsible for the majority of recent pandemics, targeting surveillance to humans, wildlife, and livestock at high-risk interfaces in these regions would be optimal (e.g., livestock farms in regions with high biodiversity). This is, intrinsically, a "One Health" approach.

However, **preventing the next pandemic** will require addressing the underlying drivers of disease emergence and will be economically, socially, and culturally challenging. Firstly, behaviors associated with a high risk of disease emergence, within EID hotspot regions, would need to be modified to reduce pandemic risk. This will be culturally and socially challenging. For example, providing alternatives to the trade in wildlife for food in parts of Southeast Asia might involve educating consumers about the relative risk of disease emergence from among wildlife, farm-raised wildlife, or domestic species. Secondly, large projects involving road building, deforestation, and dam building, as well as such economic activities as the trade in livestock and the development of intensive farms, all involve a risk of propagating a new pandemic. Efforts to deal with this risk will be economically challenging because they are likely to reduce profit (e.g., increasing surveillance for influenzas in pig and poultry farms requires funds to collect and test samples). Such efforts also present us with two opposing agendas for economic development and public health: The activities that drive emerging diseases (and result in economic loss due to disease emergence) are often critical in the economic development of the less-wealthy countries where EIDs originate.

Policy issues

Recent advances have shown that emerging diseases: (i) emerge with increasing frequency; (ii) originate in mainly tropical regions, with high wildlife biodiversity and growing human populations; (iii) are causing increasing economic impact; and (iv) once they are in the human population, rapidly gravitate to those countries with the most active travel and trade networks (e.g., countries in North America, Europe, Australia, and other high-GDP countries). The critical policy needs to develop are the following, which are particularly aligned to the Actionable Next

Steps that have emerged from the ISGP conferences concerning "One Health" and "Information Sharing":

- **A coordinated global early warning system for EIDs** that uses predictive modeling to allocate resources for surveillance to the regions most likely to propagate new pandemics (EID hotspots). Because emerging pandemics tend to cross the human-wildlife-livestock continuum, this links directly to the "One Health" Actionable Next Steps that emerged from ISGP conferences, in particular the coordination of surveillance and control across agencies. Disparate predictive modeling efforts could be coordinated by the World Health Organization (WHO)-OIE-Food and Agriculture Organization (FAO) tripartite to directly inform the regions where tripartite One Health programs are most needed. The programs proposed here should directly target surveillance of people, livestock, and wildlife at high-risk interfaces within hotspots (e.g., in and around livestock farms or extractive operations in rapidly developing, high-biodiversity countries). As proposed in the "One Health" Actionable Next Steps, this may involve partnerships among private institutions conducting predictive modeling and public institutions conducting surveillance. This effort is also aligned with "Information Sharing" Actionable Next Steps, in that the predictive modeling requires open access to data.

- **A commitment to deal with the underlying causes of pandemics by engaging a wider range of intergovernmental agencies, spanning the arenas of One Health, international development, conservation and trade.** The underlying drivers of emerging diseases include trade in wildlife and livestock, international travel, logging, and other extractive industries, as well as road-building, dam-building, and other development activities. The goal would be to deal with these underlying causes in a way that does not undermine their value to less-affluent countries. One workable solution might be for World Bank-funded development projects to be required to assess the risk of a novel EID as part of a Health Impact Assessment. Measures to deal with the risk could then be put in place as part of the funding for these projects. For example, infrastructure development projects (e.g., roads, mines, dams) in remote hotspot regions might be encouraged to provide a robust supply of safe food as an alternative to bushmeat hunting. This approach would involve engaging the United Nations Development Programme (UNDP), the International Union for Conservation of Nature (IUCN), and national agencies for international development (e.g., the United States Agency for International Development [USAID], the Australian Government Overseas Aid Program [AusAID]).

- **More accurate assessments of the cost of an EID and strategies to insure against it.** The cost of an emerging disease involves direct impacts on society, including mortality, morbidity, and the breakdown of social functioning. However, the cost of an EID often also involves other externalities that have rarely been assessed, such as the reduction in travel and trade because of the fear of future disease spread (e.g., the reduction of travel during the PDM 2009 H1N1 outbreak) or impacts on ecosystems (e.g., loss of ecosystem services due to introduced zoonoses that affect wildlife). Assessing the causes of and the economic damages due to EIDs would allow allocation of payment to deal with them. Approaches could include levying a tax on activities known to drive disease emergence. This could be an insurance approach, whereby a local government levies a fee on the private sector involved in these activities (e.g., livestock trade, road building, mining activities), or a direct payment approach wherein the cost is paid directly by governments or intergovernmental agencies. However, if the impact of pandemics is principally on countries distant to the origins of the pandemic and the location of these risky activities, it could be argued that these distant countries should also pay some form of insurance. An alternative approach would be an openly traded "EcoHealth" credit akin to the carbon credit trading approach proposed to reduce climate change.

References

Brahmbhatt, M. (2005). Avian and Human Pandemic Influenza: Economic and social impacts. (2005, November 8). Retrieved from http://www.who.int/mediacentre/events/2005/World_Bank_Milan_Brahmbhattv2.pdf

Jones, K.E., Patel, N.G., Levy, M.A., Storeygard, A., Balk, D., Gittleman, J.L., Daszak, P. (2008). Global trends in emerging infectious diseases. *Nature, 451,* 990–993.

*** A policy position paper prepared for presentation at the conference on Emerging and Persistent Infectious Diseases (EPID): Focus on the Societal and Economic Context, convened by the Institute on Science for Global Policy (ISGP) July 8–11, 2012, at George Mason University, Fairfax, Virginia.*

Figure 1. A map of global vulnerability to emerging diseases.
Image courtesy of Dr. Parviez Hosseini, senior research scientist, EcoHealth Alliance.

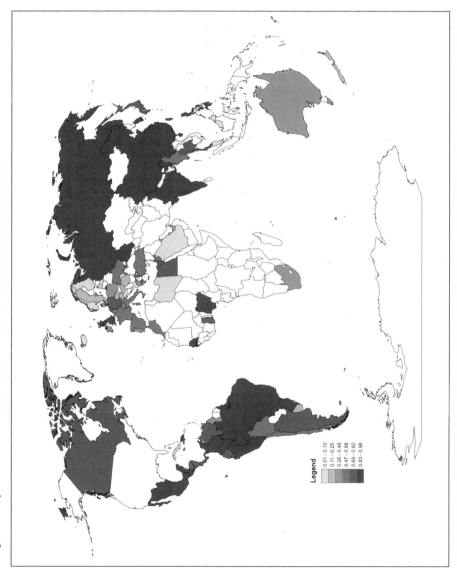

Legend
0.01 - 0.10
0.11 - 0.25
0.26 - 0.46
0.47 - 0.68
0.69 - 0.82
0.83 - 0.98

Note: This map is based on analyses in Jones et al. (2008) which show that global human activity and biodiversity are the key drivers of novel disease emergence. This map incorporates measures of global travel and trade, and countries' abilities to deal with early outbreaks and prevent them. The

Debate Summary

The following summary is based on notes recorded by the ISGP staff during the not-for-attribution debate of the policy position paper prepared by Dr. Peter Daszak (see above). Dr. Daszak initiated the debate with a 5-minute statement of his views and then actively engaged the conference participants, including other authors, throughout the remainder of the 90-minute period. This Debate Summary represents the ISGP's best effort to accurately capture the comments offered and questions posed by all participants, as well as those responses made by Dr. Daszak. Given the not-for-attribution format of the debate, the views comprising this summary do not necessarily represent the views of Dr. Daszak, as evidenced by his policy position paper. Rather, it is, and should be read as, an overview of the areas of agreement and disagreement that emerged from all those participating in the critical debate.

Debate conclusions

- Based on extensive, long-term scientific research, it is now often feasible to know the drivers that underlie the emergence of many disease pandemics, thereby greatly improving our collective ability to anticipate where and when pandemics may occur. These pandemics primarily originate in less-wealthy tropical countries characterized by extensive human activity and high biodiversity (i.e., "hotspots"). Preventing pandemics has become a "tragedy of the commons," meaning that once diseases enter the global network of human travel, they can be rapidly transmitted throughout large human populations, especially those in wealthier countries whose inhabitants travel the most.

- It remains critical that the identification of the pathogens associated with disease outbreaks be made as early as possible through efforts such as "Smart Surveillance," a global surveillance approach that targets pathogen discovery efforts in hotspot areas. While it is not currently feasible to ascertain exactly which viruses will be "bad bugs," efforts to compile a bank of sequences prior to a disease event is an important component in the development of reagents, diagnostic kits, and vaccines.

- The determination of how pandemic prevention efforts should be funded is complex, and must include governmental and private sector partnerships. A wide range of funding options needs to be researched and explored including industry taxes, direct governmental funding, and "EcoHealth" credits.

- Industries whose activities contribute to pandemic emergence must be incentivized and/or mandated to play a role in pandemic prevention efforts. Such efforts need to include implementing socially responsible practices (e.g., not building plants in hotspots and developing a system for health monitoring and pathogen discovery in employees) and potentially direct funding of pandemic prevention activities.

- Behavior change efforts that are conducted in collaboration with social scientists are key components of pandemic prevention and need to be targeted at corporations and individuals who are at risk of contracting and/or spreading disease. Since it is extremely difficult to alter human behavior that is often reflective of a society's culture, simple and low-cost solutions that address the roots of behavior need to be examined and implemented.

Current realities

During the past 60 to 80 years, approximately 10 new infectious disease events have occurred every year. Since scientific research has made it feasible to know the drivers that underlie these diseases and the potential for the associated pandemics, societies may be at a historically significant juncture with respect to their prevention. These drivers include socioeconomic factors, ecological/environmental conditions, and demographic changes. Human behavior fundamentally influences all of these drivers. Because these changes can now be tracked over time, it was contended that future changes can be anticipated, including predictions about the geographical regions where new pandemics will surface.

The majority of emerging infectious diseases and pandemics have originated within hotspots that are predominantly located in less-wealthy regions, and particularly countries in tropical areas where there is extensive human activity and high biodiversity. Once diseases enter the modern networks that characterize human travel, their increased human-to-human transmission facilitates the appearance of pandemic conditions in wealthier countries whose populations travel the most. While more-wealthy countries are susceptible to the movement of pathogens, they are also somewhat protected from the spread and detrimental impacts of waterborne pathogens (e.g., cholera) because of the infrastructure of these areas (specifically, high-quality water systems). Such protection can persist even when diseases are introduced into these populations multiple times.

While there was some disagreement about which human activities are primarily causing the appearance of pandemics, certain activities that bring animals and humans into close contact were highlighted. Many such activities are routinely pursued by businesses in less-wealthy countries that bring wildlife and humans into contact with one another (e.g., global production and trading in meat, poultry, livestock, grains, soybeans, tropical hardwoods and wildlife). These commercial programs often involve major deforestation and the construction of large farms and agricultural buildings in formerly untouched regions. These activities also require the clearing of wilderness lands for food production by poor individuals. All of these activities can significantly increase the risk that new disease pandemics appear. It was countered that this line of reasoning does not have merit because small-scale farms are epidemiologically less risky than large-scale, highly intensive farm systems.

Since the number of viruses on the planet is presently unknown, a strategy has been implemented that focuses on predicting the number of unknown viruses and estimating the cost of finding all existing viruses worldwide. While such efforts were considered manageable at a reasonable cost, it was acknowledged that it would be challenging to find funding for such a project.

The prevention of pandemics was seen as a global public good, and it was asserted that any program designed to prevent pandemics is only as strong as the "weakest link" (i.e., the weakest country's pandemic prevention strategy). Preventing pandemics was also described as a "tragedy of the commons" issue because while pandemics emerge predominantly from resource-poor countries in the tropics, they can also threaten more-wealthy countries.

Social and/or economic opportunities and challenges

Sampling every species of animal, discovering and identifying all possible viruses and pathogens, and then developing appropriate vaccines was recognized as one potentially strategic approach to pandemic prevention. While such an endeavor was seen as theoretically possible, it was viewed as untenable because of the high cost and the extensive time it would take to implement.

Instead, the implementation of "Smart Surveillance" was proposed as a lower-cost strategy to address pandemic prediction and prevention. Such a global surveillance approach would target surveillance and pathogen discovery efforts in hotspot areas where pandemics are most likely to emerge, and thus, facilitate the earlier identification of outbreaks. Specifically, it was recommended that surveillance should be targeted to the interface between humans and wildlife areas (e.g., livestock rearing on the edge of a forest) where viruses are most likely to jump the species barrier from animals to humans. Such targeted surveillance needs to be undertaken with a "One Health," multisectoral approach that brings together people from human, animal, and environmental health fields (e.g., veterinarians, medics, and ecologists).

Surveillance was considered a useful method for improving the existing knowledge base related to potentially dangerous viruses. While it is not possible to know exactly which viruses will be "bad," the bank of sequences gathered through surveillance efforts can be used to develop reagents, diagnostic kits, and vaccines in the case of a disease outbreak. Pursuing the compilation of these sequences was viewed as a priority.

Building local capacity by training people to conduct surveillance for both emerging and existing diseases was cited as an integral component of targeted surveillance. Technological limitations were viewed as a challenge to building such local surveillance capacity. For example, constant power outages may threaten the work needed to analyze samples for pathogen discovery.

It was generally agreed that efforts to change the behavior of individuals at risk of contracting and spreading disease are key components of pandemic prevention. It was recognized that since it is routinely reflective of cultural mores, efforts to change human behavior are difficult and often fail unless they address the fundamental cultural tenets. Human behavior often remains deeply rooted in emotional commitments such as the trade in wild animals as pets. Using solely educational efforts to alter human behavior was not considered especially productive. Working with social scientists to implement changes in personal behavior using simple, low-cost activities was viewed as imperative.

It was suggested that the goal of pandemic prevention is the reduction, as opposed to total control, of pandemics. Complete prevention was viewed as an unrealistic goal even if all human behavior contributing to the emergence of disease pandemics was eliminated. While most pandemics can be predicted to emerge from hotspots, a large pandemic still could appear in an area not identified as a hotspot by current mathematical models. It remains important to recognize that disease pandemics are rare events.

Confidence in predictive models for disease pandemics can be improved by conducting retrospective analyses to show how well past models have predicted events, as well as by continually testing current models and their basic assumptions "on the ground" (i.e., within hotspots). Both activities would increase the confidence policy makers have in using the results of these models for future decisions.

While it is relatively easy to discover a new virus, concern was expressed that it is challenging to predict which pathogen will be problematic (i.e., a "bad bug"). The need for research on sequences designed to predict whether a virus will become pathogenic was underscored. It was noted that the National Institute of Allergy and Infectious Diseases (NIAID) is paying attention to this type of basic viral research. Changes over time, such as increased travel and new travel routes (e.g., between Southeast Asia and Africa), were considered a barrier to predicting the risk of transmission for certain infectious diseases.

Policy issues

It was argued that the cost of halting pandemics far outweighs the financial resources necessary for prevention. It was therefore emphasized that governments need to shift their political attention as well as the allocation of human and financial resources away from reactionary approaches (e.g., vaccine development after an outbreak) toward preventive, public health courses of action. Preventive approaches are not frequently prioritized in terms of resource allocation and budgeting, and in some countries (e.g., the United States), fiscal resources allotted for public health have decreased over the years. Convincing governments to prioritize prevention was considered a major challenge. The benefits of prevention are often not recognizable since people generally do not think about events that do not occur. In addition, if an event does not take place, governments may be criticized for over-hyping a problem, which may have negative economic consequences for individuals and businesses.

Much of the discussion focused on strategies related to paying for pandemic prevention efforts, including targeted surveillance and behavior change efforts. It was proposed that the tripartite of the World Health Organization (WHO), the World Organisation for Animal Health (OIE), and the Food and Agriculture Organization of the United Nations (FAO) needs to determine the cost of surveillance and manage funding efforts.

Underlying some of these strategies was a proposal to shift responsibility for funding to certain industries. For example, one approach that was proposed and significantly debated was a tax on industry activities that contribute to pandemic emergence (e.g., the meat trade), whereby industries would be taxed in proportion to their influence on previous disease emergence as determined by insurance companies. However, it was acknowledged that to determine the allocation of payments, better economic research is needed to accurately assess the causes and economic damages of emerging infectious diseases. In addition, companies may reject the notion that they have been responsible for the emergence of diseases and request extensive proof that they are culpable.

It was questioned whether more-wealthy countries should pay taxes to prevent pandemics that are not expected to affect them (e.g., water borne diseases, such as cholera). While such diseases do not directly impact wealthier countries, there are likely downstream economic impacts from these events to more-wealthy countries (e.g., the U.S. is spending money for reconstruction in Haiti), which need to be considered.

It was generally agreed that an industry tax would be challenging to implement, and possibly untenable, due to the large amount of funds that would need to be raised to pay for pandemic prevention efforts. It was also specifically noted that convincing the public to pay taxes for another public good would be difficult to achieve. Concern was further expressed that some taxes (e.g., on meat) may disproportionately burden poor people.

As an alternative to industry funding pandemic prevention efforts, it was suggested that government agencies should directly finance prevention initiatives to allow for congressional oversight of the money. Convincing agencies to invest in these efforts will require improved cost-benefit analyses that show funding would be worthwhile. There was substantial agreement that, in places like the U.S., the cost of pandemic prevention could be offset by reallocating current resources from lower-impact diseases (e.g., Lyme Disease, rabies from bats) to pay for the prevention of disease pandemics. It was also noted that surveillance efforts are a logical extension of the U.S. Department of Defense's (DOD) current efforts, which include the building of laboratories in hotspot areas. It also was noted that some funders believe that focusing on surveillance is a "needle in a haystack" approach.

In contrast to taxes or insurance as funding mechanisms, an openly traded "EcoHealth" credit approach was also proposed. The "EcoHealth" credit was described as similar, but subtly distinct from, a carbon credit trading system. The argument was made that while carbon credits aim to stop companies from engaging in activities that inherently produce carbon, the purpose of the EcoHealth credit is not to reduce industry activities that potentially contribute to pandemic emergence (e.g., livestock production), but instead to reduce the risk of a pandemic stemming from these activities.

General consensus was expressed that industry involvement in pandemic prevention needs to include changes in industry activities that are induced through incentives, mandatory control measures, or funding provisions (e.g., from the World Bank) that make various practices compulsory. It was recommended that corporations should be incentivized or required to engage in socially responsible pandemic prevention practices, including avoiding the location of plants in hotspots, developing a health care system that includes conducting continual health monitoring and pathogen discovery on their workforces and communities, and educating employees about behavior that can prevent the spread of disease. Policies need to be implemented which mandate that large corporations conduct Health Impact Assessments to determine the potential health impact of their work prior to, during, and after project design and implementation. Such incentives could include certifying industries with a surveillance system in place as "eco-healthy." Success for these approaches will require convincing the private sector that changing their practices not only will reduce the risk of infectious disease emergence, but likely bolster profits and raise their public profile.

The importance of finding solutions that are tailored to each industry was emphasized. For instance, a certification program was identified as one method of incentivizing businesses to conduct practices that have a lower likelihood of contributing to the emergence of a disease pandemic. This example was illustrated by the PetWatch program which aims to curb wildlife practices that contribute to pandemic emergence by certifying certain wild animals sold as pets in the U.S. as "eco-healthy" if they meet certain criteria (e.g., not being shipped from an emerging disease hotspot). Consumers were considered more likely to buy pets that have this "green seal of approval" because they are captive-bred and, thus, healthier and live longer.

Hotspot surveillance was not universally viewed as the most effective mechanism for pandemic prevention. While some considered improving standards of living and wealth (which lowers people's exposure to emerging infectious diseases) a more effective route to averting pandemics, others emphasized that it is not feasible to sufficiently raise individual wealth worldwide. It was also suggested that focusing on preventing the spread of known diseases, which are easier to identify and control, is preferable to using funds to find new viruses, and that this approach will lead to a healthier population overall.

Although it was agreed that efforts to reduce the importation of infectious diseases into more-affluent countries must be strengthened, it was questioned whether building up an internal infrastructure in wealthier areas is a better use of funds than investing money in hotspots overseas. Conflicting opinions were expressed: some argued that in-country efforts would cost less and achieve a higher level of safety than hotspot surveillance while others asserted that pre-border surveillance is necessary because it is impossible to completely prevent diseases from crossing borders.

The Challenges of Implementing One Health**

Laura H. Kahn, M.D., M.P.H., M.P.P., F.A.C.P.

Research Scholar, Program on Science and Global Security
Woodrow Wilson School of Public and International Affairs
Princeton University, Princeton, New Jersey

Summary

One Health is a simple yet powerful concept: human, animal, and environmental health are inextricably linked. The goal of One Health is to integrate efforts in medicine, veterinary medicine, public health, agriculture, and environmental health (One Health Initiative, 2012). A One Health approach would prevent disease, reduce costs, improve food safety and security, and save lives. For example, potential disease outbreaks would be identified early in animals, before emerging and spreading into human populations. One Health requires disparate professions, working in diverse institutions that have distinct missions, priorities, and funding, to work together. Increasing communication and collaboration across disciplines might seem straightforward, but has proven difficult to achieve. Due to space limitations, this paper will focus on human and animal health, not environmental health. If One Health is to be achieved, the following systemic challenges must be addressed: institutions, funding, education, and jobs. Most nations do not have institutions whose primary missions are animal disease surveillance, control, and prevention. The creation of One Health organizations at the international, national, regional, and local levels, with integrated missions to improve human, animal, and environmental health, would improve global health including the prevention and control of infectious diseases. Currently, human health is vastly better funded compared with animal health (some countries have minimal or no veterinary capacity). This needs to be addressed by creating more schools of veterinary medicine, both domestically and globally. Few qualified veterinarians are pursuing careers in livestock and wildlife health, probably because limited jobs are available. Successfully implementing One Health also requires a global network of qualified individuals working locally, regionally, nationally, and internationally to share information, conduct disease surveillance in human and animal populations, monitor the environment, improve food safety and security, and communicate effectively to the public.

Current realities

The One Health approach is presently undermined by: (i) siloization in the missions of governmental and intergovernmental institutions/agencies, (ii) substantial funding differentials between human and animal health programs, and (iii) wide disparities in the education, training, and job opportunities in the human and animal health fields. In this paper, the United States will serve as the primary example to illustrate these challenges, which many nations face.

Institutions. Because the missions of institutions determine their priorities, funding, programs, and activities, human and animal health initiatives are rarely integrated with one another. For example, in the U.S., the Department of Health and Human Services' (HHS) mission is to enhance the health and well being of all Americans. Responsibility for animal health is divided across many different agencies, including the Department of Agriculture (USDA), the Department of the Interior, the Department of Commerce, the Department of Defense (DOD), and HHS. Of all these institutions involved in animal health, none have a mission statement that includes animal health. Efforts to communicate and collaborate across agencies have been difficult because of differing missions, priorities, and funding allocations.

Funding. The vast funding differences that exist between human and animal health hinder One Health implementation. For example, the Centers for Disease Control and Prevention (CDC), the federal agency responsible for public health in the U.S., has a 2013 fiscal year (FY) budget request of US$11.2 billion. The Animal and Plant Health Inspection Service (APHIS), the government entity closest to a CDC for animals, has a FY 2013 budget request of US$765 million. At the global level, the World Organisation for Animal Health (OIE) budget is miniscule (US$22 million) compared with the budgets of the World Health Organization (WHO) (US$2.3 billion) and the Food and Agriculture Organization (FAO) (US$1.2 billion), both of which are under the UN umbrella.

Education. The discrepancy in the size of human versus animal health fields, which is proportionate to the number of academic opportunities available within each field, is also an ongoing impediment to the success of One Health efforts. In the U.S., there are 137 accredited medical schools and only 28 accredited schools of veterinary medicine. Globally, medical schools outnumber veterinary medical schools by approximately 4.5 to 1, and some countries do not have any veterinary medical schools. This imbalance highlights that animal health receives less attention than human health and complicates the integration of the two communities.

Jobs. In the U.S. and globally, the ratio of practicing physicians to veterinarians is approximately 4 to 1. Most veterinarians in the U.S. pursue careers in companion animal medicine because of societal demand. There are few veterinary medical career opportunities in public health, agriculture, and wildlife management, and even fewer in biomedical research.

Social and/or economic opportunities and challenges

Funding. Discrepancies in funding extend beyond human and animal disease surveillance. There are vast funding discrepancies in biomedical research for human and animal diseases. For FY 2013, the National Institutes of Health (NIH) will fund US$29 billion for basic and clinical research for human health. The USDA's National Institute of Food and Agriculture (NIFA), the animal equivalent to the NIH, is budgeted at US$1.24 billion for FY 2013; however, no funding is budgeted specifically for research on animal health and disease. This is problematic because surveillance, control, and prevention measures depend on advances in biomedical research.

Education. Unlike medical education and training, which has traditionally received considerable federal support, veterinary medical education and training has relied primarily on state funding. States have been particularly hard hit by the 2007 global financial crisis, and schools of veterinary medicine have been struggling to stay afloat.

Jobs. The American Medical Association (AMA) asserts that there will be a critical shortage of physicians to meet future societal demands. The U.S. is already importing foreign physicians to meet its needs. According to the U.S. Bureau of Labor Statistics, position vacancies for physicians in the U.S. are expected to grow by 24% between 2010 and 2020. Because veterinarian salaries are generally lower than for physicians (while student loans can be just as high), comparatively few schools are graduating veterinarians, and thus, position vacancies for veterinarians are expected to grow by even more — 36% over the next decade. It is unclear if the anticipated positions for veterinarians will be in areas where they are most needed for One Health implementation: surveillance, control, research, and prevention in companion animal, livestock, and wildlife diseases. For example, while companion animals serve as important sentinels (particularly for toxic exposures), there are no jobs in companion animal epidemiology. Furthermore, although many deadly zoonotic diseases come from livestock and wildlife, there are few jobs in livestockor wildlife disease surveillance.

Policy issues

- **Institutions.** The creation of One Health organizations at the global, national, regional, and local levels would integrate human, animal, and environmental health as their primary mission. Leadership should be unified, allowing for more effective interdisciplinary collaboration. There are advantages and disadvantages to being an independent entity as opposed to being part of a government infrastructure. The advantages are flexibility and independence; a disadvantage is funding constraints with potentially diminished political power and legitimacy as a result. Being part of a government infrastructure improves the likelihood of long-term continuity.

- **Funding.** If a One Health organization were an independent entity, like the OIE, it would likely have a much smaller budget than if under the umbrella of a larger intergovernmental structure (like the WHO and FAO, which are agencies within the United Nations). The OIE's tiny budget, compared with the WHO and FAO budgets, illustrates this point. Funding needs to be more equitable. Policy makers must be educated about the importance of animal health and encouraged to increase animal health funding.

- **Education.** Support for both medical and veterinary medical education should be provided at the national level since funding from state or regional levels is limited. In the U.S., Medicare supports graduate medical education; a similar national funding stream should be earmarked for veterinary medical education. Education quality must be ensured through accreditation. National and international schools of public health should serve as a bridge between medicine and veterinary medicine by providing graduate degree programs in One Health. Students would study areas such as food safety and security, biodiversity and zoonotic diseases, ecosystem and environmental health, land degradation and urban development, and sustainable agriculture. Because medical, veterinary medical, and public health students are interested in global health, One Health programs would likely attract many of them to enroll.

- **Jobs.** Jobs must be created in companion animal epidemiology, as well as livestock and wildlife health, by governments, non-governmental organizations, and private industries. Jobs are currently lacking because no entity has as part of its primary mission the improvement of animal health. Policy makers must allocate funding for jobs in these areas to entice veterinary medical graduates to dedicate their careers to them.

References

National Research Council. (2005). *Animal health at the crossroads: Preventing, detecting, and diagnosing animal diseases.* Washington, D.C.: National Academies Press.

One Health Initiative. (2012). http://www.onehealthinitiative.com.

U.S. Department of Labor, Bureau of Labor Statistics. (2010). Occupational Outlook Handbook, 2009–2010. Washington, D.C.: U.S. Government Printing Office.

*** A policy position paper prepared for presentation at the conference on Emerging and Persistent Infectious Diseases (EPID): Focus on the Societal and Economic Context, convened by the Institute on Science for Global Policy (ISGP) July 8–11, 2012, at George Mason University, Fairfax, Virginia.*

Debate Summary

The following summary is based on notes recorded by the ISGP staff during the not-for-attribution debate of the policy position paper prepared by Dr. Laura Kahn (see above). Dr. Kahn initiated the debate with a 5-minute statement of her views and then actively engaged the conference participants, including other authors, throughout the remainder of the 90-minute period. This Debate Summary represents the ISGP's best effort to accurately capture the comments offered and questions posed by all participants, as well as those responses made by Dr. Kahn. Given the not-for-attribution format of the debate, the views comprising this summary do not necessarily represent the views of Dr. Kahn, as evidenced by her policy position paper. Rather, it is, and should be read as, an overview of the areas of agreement and disagreement that emerged from all those participating in the critical debate.

Debate conclusions

- Human health (e.g., infectious disease prevalence) is significantly affected by animal and environmental health. The One Health movement aims to diminish the siloization of the disciplines addressing human, animal, and environmental health by fostering collaboration among the various professional and governmental agencies. To enhance human health, the improved collaboration instituted in recent years must be built upon to cultivate more effective partnerships linking the research, regulation, and policies pertaining to humans, animals, and the environment.

- The implementation of organizational structures with specific One Health mandates, including the creation of new institutions and the reorganization of existing ones, is not the most effective route to bridging human, animal, and environmental health initiatives. Instead, One Health approaches must be encouraged within governmental agencies and societal organizations that presently focus on protecting human health.

- To garner increased support within the policy community, One Health advocates need to concentrate on empirically demonstrating (e.g., setting goals, developing metrics, and measuring outcomes) how One Health approaches improve the management of human health. Efforts centered on high-profile topics (e.g., antimicrobial resistance, Lyme disease, and raccoon rabies) can attract significant attention.

- Since taxpayers are predominantly interested in their own health and are not generally aware of the relationship between animal and human health, they are likely to be resistant to paying for animal health initiatives. One Health advocates need to frame public communication that emphasizes overall public health (wherein animal health is one component of a broader message) rather than calling attention to animal health from the outset.

- While it is important for future generations of health workers to gain an understanding of the linkages among human, animal, and environmental health, training veterinary and medical students together is not presently a realistic goal. Developing graduate courses and/or graduate degree programs related to One Health within public health schools, however, is both recommended and achievable.

Current realities

The One Health approach has been largely driven by views that both animal and environmental health significantly impact human health. A primary goal of One Health therefore has been to increase collaboration between professionals and agencies working in animal, environmental, and human health disciplines.

Animal health has been directly and indirectly correlated with human health. Direct associations have been demonstrated in terms of zoonotic diseases (i.e., animal diseases jump the species barrier and are transmitted to humans, such as influenza and antibiotic drug resistance). Indirect associations between human and animal health have also been demonstrated in terms of the relationships between human health and human wealth. For example, where animals are regarded as commodities (e.g., on farms), their well-being generates wealth that can be used to purchase good health (e.g., through the procurement of food for adequate nutrition or health services).

Throughout the 19th and early 20th centuries, there was significant collaboration between human and veterinary medical practitioners, yet a significant divide between these two branches of medicine has formed in the past century. This disengagement was attributed to a range of factors including the rise of international organizations with distinct missions and funding streams, the progression toward individual clinical care, and the separation between the education and practice of medicine and public health. It was noted, however, that some traction has been gained in the movement to develop a bridge between human and veterinary medicine, as was illustrated by the American Medical Association (AMA) House of Delegates' approval of a One Health policy resolution in 2007. The resolution solidified the AMA's commitment to working with the American Veterinary Medical Association (AVMA) on the development strategies that will enhance collaboration between the human and veterinary medical professions. Additionally, the American Academy of Pediatrics endorsed One Health in 2012.

Although the extent of present collaboration between the human and animal health fields has been considered suboptimal, examples were provided of United States agencies with mandates to protect human health that have sought to incorporate veterinarians in their work. Such agencies have included the Department of Health and Human Services (HHS), the Office of the Assistant Secretary for Preparedness and Response (ASPR), the Department of Homeland Security, and the Centers for Disease Control and Prevention (CDC). It was also noted that in 2007, the United Kingdom established a research consortium, the National Centre for Zoonosis Research (NCZR), to promote zoonoses prevention and control by building collaborations (research, training, and communication) among U.K. academics, the U.K. Health Protection Agency (HPA), and the U.K. Veterinary Laboratories Agency (VLA).

Governmental responsibilities for animal health typically have been more fragmented than governmental responsibilities for human health. For example, human health primarily has been the responsibility of HHS in the U.S., whereas the animal health domain has been distributed across agencies such as HHS, the Department of Agriculture (USDA), and the Department of the Interior (DOI), which includes the Fish and Wildlife Service. Additionally, it was noted that animal health is not included in the missions of the majority of these departments.

Institutional and agency reorganization typically has occurred during times of crisis. For example, the U.K.'s Department for Environment, Food, and Rural Affairs (DEFRA) was established in 2001 because of a perceived failure of the former Ministry of Agriculture, Fisheries, and Food (MAFF) to adequately control a serious outbreak of foot and mouth disease. Similarly, the U.S. extensively reorganized its governmental structure to create the Department of Homeland Security (DHS) following the 2001 World Trade Center and anthrax attacks.

The present post-graduate educational system reinforces the disconnect between human and animal health. Veterinary and medical schools frequently have been located on separate campuses (e.g., Cornell's College of Veterinary Medicine in Ithaca, New York, is located more than 200 miles from Cornell's Medical School in New York City), which significantly hinders cross-training and communication. The curriculum in medical schools also rarely includes animal health.

Social and/or economic opportunities and challenges

It was asserted that the disparate missions, priorities, and funding sources of both international institutions and national agencies have been significant barriers to the implementation of One Health initiatives because siloization has the potential to engender narrow organizational purviews that do not inherently bridge the central issues pertaining to human, animal, and environmental health.

The One Health movement has been hindered by its advocates' concentration on garnering broad support across the scientific and policy communities for sweeping institutional and funding changes based predominantly on the platform that human, animal, and environmental health are inextricably linked. While the success of the present approach has been limited, an opportunity exists for the movement to gain traction by refocusing its efforts toward demonstrating the value of One Health for specific infectious disease problems through deliverable-driven initiatives. The potential effectiveness of this tactic was exemplified by the history of the public health movement, where proven achievements for specific health interventions in the late 19th and early 20th centuries have been considered instrumental to fostering support for public health efforts.

Due to the well-documented correlations between economics (e.g., individual income and/or gross domestic product) and health status, the "One Wealth" concept (i.e., more equitable wealth distribution) may be more effective than One Health as an avenue for improving global health. Yet, it was also argued that One Health may present an opportunity to simultaneously improve the wealth and health of individuals. For example, the World Bank explicitly supported One Health principles for the control of zoonotic diseases in its 2012 "People, Pathogens and Our Planet, Volume 2" report. The World Bank noted that (i) economic losses stemming from six major zoonotic disease outbreaks between 1997–2009 totaled approximately US$80 billion, (ii) the estimated avoided losses would have averaged US$6.7 billion per year if these outbreaks had been prevented, and (iii) One Health approaches could potentially provide efficiency gains by either conducting more activities with the same resources or conducting the same amount of activities with fewer resources. Additionally, it was noted that animal health is a strong contributor to human wealth in many nations (particularly in less-affluent regions).

Although it was acknowledged that augmenting interprofessional education programs between veterinary and medical students would be valuable, it was also noted that this goal would be extremely difficult to achieve because of entrenched attitudes toward higher education organizational structures and the existing emphasis on individual health within medical schools. While bridging veterinary and medical schools was viewed as impractical, an opportunity exists to connect human and animal disciplines through public health. As in medical school curricula, animal health issues largely have been absent from public health curricula. However, an intrinsic commonality exists between veterinary medicine and public health because both are population-based disciplines. The development of graduate courses and/or graduate degree programs related to One Health within public health schools can be a constructive starting point for educating a future generation of practitioners on the intersection between human and animal health.

Because national agencies and intergovernmental organizations rarely have directives that focus strictly on animal health, garnering funding for animal health initiatives (even when the end goal is to improve human health) was considered a significant challenge. While it was suggested that the creation of an overarching One Health institution, in which human, animal, and environment departments are structured under a One Health umbrella, would make the distribution of resources more equitable, such reorganization does not always simplify funding streams. Even within unified institutions funding is frequently problematic because internal divisions still compete for budget allocations and "turf wars" often develop.

Policy issues

There was general consensus that the basic concepts underlying the One Health approach are important for the protection of human health. Although some collaboration among the environmental, animal, and human health communities has already begun, the targeted expansion of the present cooperation among these groups, in which collaborations are based on specific deliverables, would ultimately benefit human health.

However, policy makers generally do not change their *modus operandi* unless a specific objective is presented to them with a strategic plan for how to achieve that goal. A greater emphasis needs to be placed on empirically demonstrating through such means as setting goals, developing metrics, and measuring outcomes, how One Health approaches improve the way that human health is managed. There was general agreement that this targeted approach would gain greater traction than providing policy makers information on funding and/or job shortages within the animal health community.

With respect to providing policy makers with goals, plans, and deliverables, the One Health community needs to focus its efforts on several high-profile topics to garner increased attention. Suggestions of substantive areas that policy makers would likely be interested in included antimicrobial resistance as a function of agricultural practices, Lyme disease, and raccoon rabies.

Although it has been widely acknowledged within the scientific community that animal health has the capacity to acutely impact human health, taxpayers often are not aware of this relationship and are primarily interested in their own health. Because taxpayers may resist paying for animal health initiatives, One Health advocates need to frame their public communications in ways that emphasize overall public health, treating animal health as one component of a broader message rather than calling attention to animal health from the outset. It was emphasized that the end goal of changing the message would be to achieve greater support for the intersection of animal and human health in a way that effectively influences the taxpayers who, in turn, influence decisions made by policy makers.

The view that significant institutional changes are needed to establish structures with specific mandates for One Health, either through the creation of new institutions or the reorganization of existing ones, was strongly contested. Although the disparate missions, priorities, and funding of the present institutional system has complicated efforts to bring One Health to the forefront of agendas, the general consensus was that collaborative efforts that bridge human, animal, and environmental health needs can be achieved through other routes that do not require such extreme institutional reform. Additionally, it was argued that restructuring existing institutions would be exceptionally difficult to achieve given that many have long histories, would be resistant to change, and have primary responsibilities that far exceed the scope of One Health.

While strong sentiments were generally expressed against the creation of new institutions for One Health, a caveat was proposed that received support. It was suggested that new countries (e.g., South Sudan), or countries that are presently undergoing significant reorganization due to financial crises (e.g., Greece), may be more receptive to establishing an organizational structure where human, animal, and environmental health are brought together in a holistic manner. If such efforts prove to be successful (e.g., streamlining the efficiency of government, reducing costs, and effectively solving human health problems), other governments may then be incentivized to implement similar changes.

Will a Comprehensive Global Source Attribution System Provide for Cost-Effective Food Safety?**

Gay Y. Miller, D.V.M., Ph.D.Professor, Department of Veterinary Pathobiology, College of Veterinary Medicine, and Adjunct Professor, Department of Agriculture and Consumer Economics, College of Agricultural and Environmental Sciences, University of Illinois, Urbana, Illinois

Summary

We are in a globalization era that includes increased demands for food and food safety. Food chains are comprised of complex networks of people and companies, as well as the movement of raw ingredients and food components. In the United States, PulseNet already creates a genetic fingerprint of organisms suspected to cause foodborne illness; however, the source of most outbreaks is never identified. It is unclear how much of this food safety challenge can be rectified by a surveillance system that is deeper (i.e., has a more thorough collection of data), more general (i.e., collects data across a wider range of production systems), and adds data from different sources (e.g., from animal, animal feeds, and food sampling). While more research is needed, a focus on infrastructure improvements will result in the largest marginal benefit to food safety, with higher cost effectiveness than a global surveillance system. The Actionable Next Steps emerging from ISGP conferences focus primarily on improving global surveillance. This focus needs to be balanced against, and possibly superseded by, considerations related to infrastructure improvements and food safety prevention. Most importantly, Actionable Next Steps to prevent and mitigate foodborne illness should include a focus on the preventive components of the U.S. Food and Drug Administration's (FDA) Food Safety Modernization Act (FSMA), the most extensive reform of the U.S. food safety laws in 70 years.

Current realities

Since we are in a globalization era, high-speed transportation and communications have provided incredible opportunities for trade, resulting in an expanding and more efficient global economy that can positively affect many societies. But enhanced economies come with costs, including increased potential for disease transmission of exotic/invasive species; greater use of fossil fuels, contributing to environmental change and potential degradation; and populations desiring higher quality and quantities of food and water. As the world becomes increasingly globalized, a large portion of the global population is also at increased risk of foodborne illness — namely, the very young, the very old, and the immuno-compromised. Consumer practices, such as meals eaten away from home and the purchase of more table-ready or quick-preparation food products, place an increasing responsibility for food safety outside the direct control of the consumer. Thus, consumer desire for external food safety oversight and control is greater than in the past. In addition, political instabilities and long-standing animosities may be linked to bioterrorism and potentially, may lead to intentional food adulteration. Risks for bioterrorism are difficult to assess. Once a particular food is categorized as low risk, it may be monitored less or differently, and thus, the vulnerability to hazards from this food increases.

Food chains are comprised of complex networks of people, companies, and the movement of raw ingredients and food components. Specializations (e.g., refinements and simplifications of tasks) at many levels in food production allow for increasing the size of production systems and facilities, which also increases the potential for wider scale and scope of food safety problems. Yet, specializations also stimulate improvements in food safety by decreasing accidental contaminations or errors leading to outbreaks. Agricultural production is occurring on larger farms and food processing is occurring in larger plants, farther from the points of consumption.

The continuous occurrences of catastrophic events (e.g., food-related outbreaks or environmental disasters) frequently cause agencies to respond primarily to areas that are considered urgent in the short-term, rather than to address those issues that are considered important in the long-term. Such a trend undermines the effectiveness of how agencies can prevent and/or mitigate foodborne illness. Personnel time tends to be used more to manage crises (e.g., the 2011 radiation contamination event in Japan or Deepwater Horizon), than for making decisions involving the underlying scientific and economic factors associated with the catastrophes. Catastrophes also influence funding levels and the stability of programs. The FSMA aims to ensure that the U.S. food supply is safe by shifting the focus from response to the prevention of contamination and by requiring prevention accountability.

The FSMA requires imported food, which comprises a substantial percentage of foods consumed in the U.S., to be as safe as domestically produced food. The shift toward prevention comes with a cost, however. Economic efficiency suggests such costs be borne by the beneficiaries. Funding for the FSMA would be borne primarily by the food industry and therefore, indirectly, by consumers.

There is, of course, value in the surveillance of foods and the early detection of foodborne illness. PulseNet, a national network of public health and food regulatory agency laboratories coordinated by the U.S. Centers for Disease Control and Prevention (CDC), already captures human, environmental, and investigation samples. Standardized molecular subtyping using pulsed-field gel electrophoresis (PFGE) is used on these samples to create a genetic fingerprint of organisms suspected to have caused foodborne illness; however, it remains difficult for the U.S. to solve outbreaks currently identified by PulseNet since the source of most outbreaks is never identified.

Social and/or economic opportunities and challenges

In the U.S., the legal authority needed to implement the Actionable Next Steps emerging from ISGP conferences exists through the FSMA. The FDA is currently studying ways to quickly trace foods back to a common contamination that leads to foodborne illness based on a system that is practical, feasible, and rapid. The FSMA also gives the FDA broad authority to provide foreign countries assistance for improving the food safety of products exported to the U.S., including risk-based inspections. However, most foodborne illness outbreaks currently remain unsolved. The ISGP Actionable Next Steps suggest this challenge would be rectified by the development of a surveillance system that is deeper, more general, and adds more data from different sources. In addition, they recommend the expansion of a PulseNet-style identification approach, both within the U.S. and globally. It is unclear, however, how much these recommendations would help in identifying foodborne illness outbreaks.

The benefits and costs of implementing food safety surveillance, compared with a combination of enhanced food safety infrastructure and practices, as well as the relative value of focusing on environmental issues (e.g., enhancing basic water quality), especially in less wealthy nations, are generally unknown. While several case studies have identified the needs related to certain foodborne illnesses in specific less-wealthy countries, it is difficult to extrapolate these results to other countries. Each country has a unique history, set of circumstances, and problems, all of which influence the factors that might improve their food safety. Although further studies are needed, a focus on infrastructure improvements will result in the largest marginal benefit to food safety, with lower costs than those anticipated in establishing an improved global surveillance system. Specifically, current good management practices (GMP) exist that are Hazard Analysis and Critical Control Points (HACCP) linked and identified at each step of the food chain. Indeed, the FSMA suggests that GMPs will be the foundation of preventive practices. The

FSMA will combine the basic elements learned from GMPs with a certification process ensuring their use.

Policy issues

The Actionable Next Steps distributed by the ISGP focus solely on global surveillance. This focus needs to be balanced against, and possibly superseded by, considerations related to infrastructure improvements and food safety prevention, including a focus on the preventive components of the FSMA.

- Agencies like the FDA should place more emphasis on the preventive components of FSMA, namely "Title I — Improving Capacity to Prevent Food Safety Problems," which aims to improve the capacity to prevent food safety problems through governance on aspects of food safety including the registration of food facilities, standards for produce safety, and sanitary transportation of food. Next in importance, agencies should emphasize "Title III — Improving the Safety of Imported Food" of the FSMA, which focuses on decreasing foodborne illness risks from imported foods by helping to build food safety capacity of governments, combined with supplier verification and inspections.

- Efforts in food-exporting countries should focus on infrastructural changes that broadly enhance the safety of food and water. Environmental interventions aimed at foodborne illness prevention will result in larger, more cost-effective improvements in food safety than will implementation of a global surveillance system that focuses on responding to food safety problems one-by-one as they arise. Developing a global surveillance system that can and will be used to divert or shut off exports (to the U.S. or elsewhere) is inefficient and excessively forceful.

- Research is needed to: (i) identify the benefits and costs of food safety improvements for different countries, and (ii) examine the relative importance of food safety surveillance, compared with enhancing infrastructure and improving food safety practice and quality, for countries exporting foods.

- To improve surveillance, PulseNet needs to also sample animals, animal feeds, and foods.

- Exciting consumer educational programming should be developed that includes information on the farm-to-fork spectrum and improved food safety practices. These educational programs should be developed and funded through public-private partnerships.

The potential social and economic issues associated with implementing these Actionable Next Steps are the same as for the recommendations proposed above, which include:

- **Social impact.** Improved food safety practices may lead to targeted blame for deaths or illnesses, which may have social and psychological implications (e.g., guilt) for food production firms.

- **Economic impact.** Improving food safety preventive practices and surveillance may result in an increased cost of foods, food production, and food processing; the economic gain of these improvements (e.g., a decrease in health care costs and mortality) is unknown.

- **Potential for loss of small-scale producers/processors.** Although the FSMA supports small businesses (e.g., through exemptions), small businesses identified as the source of a foodborne illness outbreak will be challenged to survive the associated effects (e.g., litigation). Costs of implementing GMP and surveillance efforts will also lead to decreased net incomes of small-scale food producers (especially in less-wealthy nations).

References

Prüss-Üstün, A., & Corvalán, C. (2007). How much disease burden can be prevented by environmental interventions? *Epidemiology, 18*(1), 167–178.

The New FDA Food Safety Modernization Act (FSMA). (2011). Retrieved April 4, 2012, from http://www.fda.gov/Food/FoodSafety/FSMA.

*** A policy position paper prepared for presentation at the conference on Emerging and Persistent Infectious Diseases (EPID): Focus on the Societal and Economic Context, convened by the Institute on Science for Global Policy (ISGP) July 8–11, 2012, at George Mason University, Fairfax, Virginia.*

Debate Summary

The following summary is based on notes recorded by the ISGP staff during the not-for-attribution debate of the policy position paper prepared by Dr. Gay Miller (see above). Dr. Miller initiated the debate with a 5-minute statement of her views and then actively engaged the conference participants, including other authors, throughout the remainder of the 90-minute period. This Debate Summary represents the ISGP's best effort to accurately capture the comments offered and questions posed by all participants, as well as those responses made by Dr. Miller. Given the not-for-attribution format of the debate, the views comprising this summary do not necessarily represent the views of Dr. Miller, as evidenced by her policy position paper. Rather, it is, and should be read as, an overview of the areas of agreement and disagreement that emerged from all those participating in the critical debate.

Debate conclusions

- The emphasis of efforts to improve food safety through the prevention of foodborne diseases need to be shifted from a reactionary to a proactive approach. By developing strong preventive measures that reduce the number of hazards in the food supply, the food safety system can be significantly strengthened.

- The United States has made considerable progress in establishing and supporting legislation that promotes prudent preventive measures across the food supply chain. The U.S. Food and Drug Administration's (FDA) Food Safety Modernization Act (FSMA) focuses heavily on hazard prevention through the creation of a regulatory framework that includes mandatory preventive controls for food facilities, mandatory produce safety standards, and authority to prevent intentional contamination. While some of the ambitious aims delineated in FSMA will be challenging to achieve, there is significant potential for FSMA to improve food safety.

- Global surveillance, including traceback and source attribution, is a critical component of both improved foodborne disease prevention and efforts to effectively respond to foodborne disease outbreaks. Accurate data are essential to identify where changes in the food supply chain can be made to avert future disease outbreaks and to halt disease transmission when outbreaks occur.

- The globalization of the food supply has rapidly increased the proportion of food that is imported by most countries. Although inspections of imported food items are essential components of overall food safety strategies, it is not economically viable or practically feasible to rely solely on this approach. Ensuring that food safety practices in export countries are consistent with accepted food safety standards in import countries (e.g., the U.S.) is essential.

- Since the actual health risks from foodborne diseases often differ significantly from the public's perceptions of these risks, establishing acceptable levels of food safety is difficult. Such uncertainty also complicates setting publicly acceptable policy goals and the effectiveness of public messaging concerning foodborne diseases.

Current realities

The complex web of establishments that comprise the global food supply chain include farms, processors, manufacturers, distributors, grocers, and restaurants. Examples were provided related to the many ways that food may become contaminated with pathogenic organisms at different points along the food supply chain. With respect to farms, it was noted that both produce and animals are inherently susceptible to disease-causing microorganisms because produce is grown in dirt (which naturally harbors microorganisms, such as *Listeria*, that may be pathogenic to humans) and animals are raised in close contact with one another (which promotes the spread of microbes that may be pathogenic to humans and/ or animals). Food may also become contaminated through certain methods used in processing plants (e.g., cooling hundreds of poultry carcasses together in ice water baths). Additionally, human error in handling (e.g., not washing hands before touching food items) or preparation (e.g., inappropriate cooking times or temperatures) may also contaminate food with pathogenic microbes in grocery stores, restaurants, or homes.

A considerable proportion of the food consumed in the U.S. is imported from foreign countries. It was estimated that approximately 80% of the seafood, 30% of the fruits and nuts, and 15% of the vegetables eaten by Americans has been imported from overseas. International trade has significantly complicated efforts to protect consumers from foodborne illnesses.

Good Agricultural Practices (GAP) and Good Manufacturing Practices (GMP) were considered critical to ensuring food safety. It was contended that although the majority of companies, especially large companies that have significant resources, conduct GAP and GMP, lapses in these practices can result in outbreaks of foodborne diseases.

The U.S. FDA's Food Safety Modernization Act (FSMA), signed into law in 2011, was created to better protect the health of Americans by strengthening the food safety system. A critical priority of FSMA has been to shift attention toward preventing the contamination or adulteration of food rather than focusing on reacting to food safety problems as they arise. The preventive component of FSMA centers on mandatory preventive controls for food facilities, mandatory produce safety standards, and authority to prevent intentional contamination.

Molecular subtyping (i.e., "fingerprinting") of foodborne disease-causing bacteria has been increasingly performed both for traceback and to facilitate the early identification of common sources of outbreaks. In the U.S., the FDA has used molecular sequencing of isolates coming from foods and processing plants to identify the source of outbreaks. Additionally, PulseNet (a national network of public health and food regulatory agency laboratories coordinated by the Centers for Disease Control and Prevention [CDC]) has developed a national, electronic database of DNA fingerprints that can be searched for human isolates to link seemingly sporadic cases of foodborne diseases. Although molecular databases such as PulseNet are limited by the amount of information present at any given time within their library of data, they have significantly evolved during the past few years. Such databases will continue to grow stronger as more disease-causing bacteria isolated from humans and from suspected food are fingerprinted and entered into computer catalogs.

Social and/or economic opportunities and challenges

Because naturally occurring microorganisms (both harmful and innocuous) are highly prevalent on farms, it was contended that specifically targeting animal or produce farms to reduce pathogens in food is an impractical, and potentially unattainable, solution. This viewpoint was called into question with evidence of successful interventions at the farm-level. It was highlighted that both Sweden and Denmark have significantly reduced *Salmonella* in humans (now less than 1% in Sweden) by implementing control programs that heavily focus on monitoring herds and flocks and eliminating infected animals on poultry and pig farms. While scientific literature has conclusively demonstrated that the methods employed in Sweden and Denmark have succeeded, the costs associated with these practices may limit the ability of other countries to duplicate their programs.

Because the food supply has become increasingly globalized, ensuring that food safety practices in export countries are consistent with accepted standards in the U.S. has been recognized as critically important. The recent FSMA legislation has enhanced the FDA's authority to ensure that imported products are considered safe for U.S. consumers by strengthening existing and establishing new priorities for various issues, including (i) importer accountability, (ii) third-party certification, (iii) certification for high-risk foods, (iv) a voluntary qualified importer program, and (v) authority to deny entry. While the FSMA initiatives related to food importation were viewed as positive steps, concerns were expressed that many of these aims will be extremely difficult to achieve. For example, it was noted that FSMA requires the FDA to at least double foreign facility inspections in each of the next five years (i.e., raising the number of inspections from approximately 600 in 2011 to 19,000 in 2016). Given the high costs associated with foreign facility inspections and the current economic climate, it was considered highly unlikely that the FDA will be able to fulfill this particular objective.

It was contended that cost-effectively improving food safety is a "wicked problem" (i.e., a complex problem in which incomplete, contradictory, and/or changing requirements are such that each attempted solution often seems to create a new problem). While it was acknowledged that protecting consumers is an arduous task, and that the risk of foodborne diseases can never be completely removed, it was also emphasized that many positive steps can be taken to improve food safety. For instance, it was noted that there are numerous activities and interventions that have been proven to reduce food contamination (e.g., GAP, GMP, sanitation, storage temperature, and consumer handling practices) that can be better implemented. Additionally, it was contended that existing technological solutions (e.g., irradiation) and the potential development of new technological solutions (e.g., smart packaging to detect when food goes bad) can provide alternative ways to further strengthen the safety of the food supply.

Due to inherent ambiguities in the concept of risk, determining what constitutes reasonable levels of food safety was considered a significant challenge. While risk assessors and regulators have attempted to determine acceptable levels of risk for several decades, it has been repeatedly demonstrated that risk perceptions and actual risk vastly differ across societal spheres (e.g., whether someone is rich or poor, resides in a more- or less-affluent country, and is healthy or immuno-compromised). These views also vary depending on the context within which they are considered (e.g., higher risks, such as those associated with cancer drugs, may be tolerated when the potential benefit is perceived to be sizable). Such uncertainty complicates efforts to set food safety goals and makes public messages difficult to effectively construct.

Sanitation issues in less-affluent countries, such as poor-quality irrigation water, have been identified as a significant concern for food safety related to fresh produce. Developing the infrastructure for items such as enhanced water quality is costly, time-consuming, and difficult to achieve. It was therefore emphasized that sanitation improvements must be viewed as just one component of long-term food safety strategies.

Policy issues

Preventing hazards from entering the food supply was emphasized as the most effective route to improving food safety. While there are many activities that can be considered preventive measures, the discussion primarily focused on the preventive components of FSMA and global surveillance.

Prevention is the cornerstone of FSMA and the act sets a high bar for the global food industry to reduce the contamination of food products. Due to the complexity of the food system (i.e., the many points along the food supply chain where contamination can occur) and the changing nature of the food supply (e.g., the rapidly increasing volume of imports), successfully implementing FSMA will not be straightforward. Despite the expected challenges, it was acknowledged that there is significant potential for FSMA to improve food safety in the U.S., as well as within countries that export to the U.S.

Significant debate stemmed from the viewpoint that surveillance may not produce a considerable return on investment because most food production industries already know which process areas are problematic within the food chain and what organisms must be monitored to prevent diseases outbreaks. While it was acknowledged that the food industry and regulatory agencies are frequently aware of which pathogens contribute to foodborne diseases in a population, it was asserted that the vehicles (i.e., food products) are often unknown. Linking a disease outbreak to the food that is the source of contamination can be challenging, but to effectively improve the food safety within the industry, efforts must be made to accurately identify the sources of foodborne diseases.

Because microbes are naturally present on farms, concern was expressed that the surveillance activities of traceback and source attribution will predominantly establish farms as the origin of foodborne diseases, even when good agricultural practices are exercised. This emphasis can lead to punitive actions that would be especially detrimental to smaller farms. The primary goals of traceback and source attribution, however, are not focused on punishing farms (or manufacturing companies), but are to enable effective responses that halt transmission when outbreaks occur and to identify where changes can be made to avert future problems.

Given that traceback and source attribution are frequently employed after a foodborne disease outbreak has occurred, uncertainty was expressed regarding whether these surveillance activities can significantly contribute to the prevention of food safety problems. However, a mindset shift is needed wherein traceback and source attribution are considered critical components of prevention programs. Transmission containment (i.e., the prevention of additional cases of a particular foodborne disease) depends on accurate data for the rapid identification of where contamination occurred within the food supply chain and/or which food was the vehicle of infection. This was exemplified by the chain of events related to a past outbreak of *E. Coli* O157:H7 associated with raw cookie dough. Although eggs were considered the most likely origin of contamination, source attribution demonstrated that flour was the actual cause. Once flour was established as the vehicle, the cookie dough producer began using pasteurized flour and was thereby able to prevent future cases of *E. Coli* O157:H7.

Source attribution data can also be prospectively used to evaluate the impact of interventions. It was noted that this application of source attribution data is currently being performed in the United Kingdom for Campylobacteriosis. Campylobacteriosis, which can stem from different animal reservoirs, is the most commonly reported bacterial cause of infectious intestinal disease in England and Wales and has been estimated to cost the economy approximately GBP£1.5 billion pounds. A program in the U.K. has employed multilocus sequence typing to develop a baseline for sources of Campylobacteriosis, and is currently implementing experiments in the poultry industry in an effort to control the disease, and then evaluate whether the attribution of animal reservoir to human disease changes as a result of those interventions.

Only a small proportion of the food that is globally consumed has been inspected. Although inspections were considered useful components of overall food safety strategies, it was argued that a wholesale reliance on inspections is neither economically viable nor feasible.

Government agencies responsible for minimizing the risks associated with food consumption need to strengthen their engagement with consumer groups to understand and address their concerns. Efforts must be made to ensure that both sides recognize that negotiating acceptable levels of risk may be neither practical nor beneficial given that risk perceptions substantially vary within and between societies.

Acknowledgment

Numerous individuals and organizations have made important contributions to the Institute on Science for Global Policy (ISGP) program on Emerging and Persistent Infectious Diseases (EPID). Some of these contributions directly supported the efforts needed to organize and convene the invitation-only ISGP conference on *EPID: Focus on the Societal and Economic Context* held at the George Mason University in Fairfax, Virginia, July 8-11, 2012. Other contributions aided the ISGP in preparing the material presented in this book, including not only the eight invited policy position papers, but a record, without attribution, of the views presented in the discussions, critical debates, and caucuses that ensued.

We would like to thank our colleagues at the George Mason University, and especially Dr. Roger Stough, Vice President for Research, and Mr. Kerry Bolognese, Vice President for Federal Relations, for their many contributions toward the success of this conference. The level of cooperation and support from our George Mason University colleagues set an exceptionally high standard and was greatly appreciated.

The process underlying all ISGP conferences began with the recognition that EPID and related aspects of Food Safety and Security (FSS) and Synthetic Biology (SB) are topics that deserve significantly greater attention from both domestic and international policy makers. The willingness of those in the scientific and policy communities who have expertise and experience with EPID, FSS, and SB to be interviewed by the ISGP staff was a critical early step in creating and updating the Strategic Roadmap on EPID. The resultant Strategic Roadmap describes the two-year-plus series of ISGP conferences focused on different policy aspects of EPID, FSS, and SB. The support for the EPID Strategic Roadmap by the governments engaged with the ISGP was the basis for convening a series of three conferences focused on different aspects of these broad fields. A list of ISGP conferences on EPID, FSS, and SB is provided below.

The efforts of the scientific presenters invited by the ISGP in both preparing policy position papers and engaging policy makers in the vigorous debates and caucuses that comprised these conferences were especially appreciated. Their biographies are provided in each of the ISGP books published following each conference (ISGP books are available to the public and can be downloaded from the ISGP Web site: www.scienceforglobalpolicy.org)

The implementation of the largely scientific and technological recommendations emerging from the previous four ISGP conferences need to be evaluated in terms of their societal, economic, and ethical impact on the public. Thus, the ISGP invited eight highly distinguished subject-matter experts working on social, behavioral, economic, and ethical topics to prepare the policy position papers addressed at the ISGP conference convened at George Mason University. These presenters were asked to prepare their policy position papers in response to four areas of consensus and their related actionable next steps that collectively summarize all the earlier recommendations. This summary of the earlier recommendations was prepared by the ISGP and is presented as part of the Introduction to this book.

The success of all ISGP programs critically depends on the active engagement of all participants in the often-intense debates that originate among the scientific presenters, the subject-matter experts, and policy makers. The audience, invited by the ISGP after consultation with a variety of participating governments and organizations, provides an outstanding level of discussion focused on enhancing and expanding the general understanding. The exchange of strongly held views, innovative proposals, and critiques generated from questions and debates fosters an unusual, even unique, environment focused on clarifying understanding for the nonspecialist. These debates and caucuses addressed specific questions related to formulating and implementing effective public policy pertaining to EPID, FSS, and SB. The exchanges at the George Mason University conference were especially valuable in identifying the societal, economic, and ethical issues attendant to implementing the scientifically credible options that emerged from earlier ISGP conferences on EPID, FSS, and/or SB.

The ISGP is greatly indebted to all those who participated in these vigorous, not-for-attribution debates and caucuses.

The ISGP Board of Directors also deserves special thanks for their time and efforts made in creating a vital and growing not-for-profit organization. The current membership of the ISGP Board of Directors and their brief biographical background are presented at the end of this book.

The energetic, highly professional work of the ISGP staff merits special acknowledgment. Their outstanding interviewing, organizing, and writing skills were essential to recording the often-diverse views and perspectives expressed in the critical debates, capturing the areas of consensus and next steps from the caucuses, and persevering through the extensive editing process needed to assure the accuracy of the material published here. All of their work is gratefully acknowledged. Their biographies are provided in this book.

The U.S. Department of Health and Human Services (HHS), the U.S. Department of State (DOS), and the U.S. Department of Homeland Security (DHS) are acknowledged as the co-sponsors of this work, under a 'work for others' arrangement between the U.S. Department of Health and Human Services and ISGP.

Finally, the ISGP expresses sincere appreciation for the advice and financial support of the National Intelligence Council. Major scientific and financial support was also provided by the Istituto Regionale di Ricerca in Milan, Italy. The ISGP also benefited from the recommendations and generous gifts provided by the MARS Corp., Novartis, GlaxoSmithKline, and Mr. Edward Bessey. The ISGP gratefully acknowledges the ongoing support provided by the Critical Path Institute, the University of Arizona, and the University of Minnesota.

Dr. George H. Atkinson
Founder and Executive Director
Institute on Science for Global Policy
September 9, 2012

ISGP conferences on Emerging and Persistent Infectious Diseases:

- EPID: Global Perspectives, convened Dec. 6–9, 2009 in Tucson, Arizona, U.S.

- EPID: Focus on Surveillance, convened Oct. 17–20, 2010 in Warrenton, Virginia, U.S.

- EPID: Focus on Prevention, convened June 5–8, 2011 in San Diego, California, U.S.

- EPID: Focus on Mitigation, convened Oct. 23–26, 2011 in Edinburgh, Scotland, U.K.

Biographical information of scientific presenters

Prof. Arthur Caplan, Ph.D.

Prof. Arthur Caplan, a renowned bioethicist, is the Drs. William F and Virginia Connolly Mitty Professor, and head of the Division of Bioethics at New York University Langone Medical Center in New York City. Prior to this, he was the Sidney D. Caplan Professor of Bioethics at the University of Pennsylvania, where he held various positions from 1994 until July 2012. Before joining University of Pennsylvania, Prof. Caplan taught at the University of Minnesota, the University of Pittsburgh, and Columbia University. A prolific writer, Prof. Caplan is the author or editor of more than 30 books and 550 peer-reviewed papers, and connects with the public through several popular media outlets, including his column on bioethics for MSNBC.com. Prof. Caplan has served on numerous national and international committees including the National Cancer Institute Biobanking Ethics Working Group, the Advisory Committee to the United Nations on Human Cloning and the Presidential Advisory Committee on Gulf War Veterans' Illnesses. In addition, Prof. Caplan is currently the ethics adviser to the Department of Defense/Defense Advanced Research Projects Agency (DARPA) on synthetic biology. Prof. Caplan is the recipient of several awards, including the McGovern Medal of the American Medical Writers Association, the Franklin Award from the City of Philadelphia, and the 2011 Patricia Price Browne Prize in Biomedical Ethics.

Dr. Peter Daszak, Ph.D.

Dr. Peter Daszak is President of the EcoHealth Alliance, a global organization dedicated to innovative conservation science linking ecology and the health of humans and wildlife. A disease ecologist in the field of conservation medicine, Dr. Daszak's research has been instrumental in identifying and predicting the impact of emerging diseases across the globe. In his prior role as Executive Vice President of Health at EcoHealth Alliance, Dr. Daszak directed a program of collaborative research, education, and conservation policy, which examined, among other things, the role of wildlife trade in disease introduction and the emergence of novel zoonotic viruses lethal to humans. He joined EcoHealth Alliance in 2001 as Executive Director of its Consortium for Conservation Medicine (the first formal interinstitutional partnership bringing conservation and disease ecology under one umbrella). Dr. Daszak is a member of the Institute of Medicine's (IOM) Forum on Microbial Threats and served on the IOM Committee on global surveillance for emerging zoonoses, the National Research Council committee on the future of veterinary research, and the International Standing Advisory Board of the Australian Biosecurity CRC. He has authored more than 150 papers, and his work has been the focus of extensive media coverage ranging from popular press articles to television appearances. He received the 2000 CSIRO Medal from Australia's Commonwealth Scientific and Industrial Research Organisation for collaborative research and is Editor-in-Chief of the Springer journal EcoHealth.

Dr. Vanessa Hayes, Ph.D.

Dr. Vanessa Hayes is Professor of Genomic Medicine at the J. Craig Venter Institute in San Diego. Prior to joining the Venter Institute in 2010, Dr. Hayes headed a genetics laboratory focused on the genetic basis of HIV susceptibility in local populations at the University of Stellenbosch, Cape Town, South Africa, and was group leader of the Cancer Genetics research group at both the Garavan Institute of Medical Research and the Children's Cancer Institute in Australia. Dr. Hayes' work focuses on defining the extent of human genome diversity and how this diversity impacts human health. She is also a proponent of information sharing, particularly with respect to genetic sequences. In 2010, she made headlines by co-leading a study to define the extent of human diversity by generating the genome sequence of South African Noble Peace Laureate Archbishop Desmond Tutu, and a Bushman (hunter-gatherer) from the Kalahari region of Namibia. Published in Nature in 2010, this work was the first genome sequence of an indigenous person. Dr. Hayes is the recipient of numerous awards, including a Fulbright Australian-American Professional Scholarship, the Ruth Stephens Gani Medal for Human Genetics and the New South Wales Premier's Award for Outstanding Cancer Research. She has also been appointed as an Honorary Professor of Medical Sciences at the rural-based University of Limpopo, South Africa.

Dr. Laura H. Kahn, M.D., M.P.H., M.P.P.

Dr. Laura H. Kahn is a Physician and Research Scholar with the Program on Science and Global Security at the Woodrow Wilson School of Public and International Affairs, Princeton University, with expertise in public health, biodefense, and pandemics. Before joining Princeton in 2002, she was Managing Physician for the New Jersey Department of Health and Senior Services, and a Medical Officer for the U.S. Food and Drug Administration. In 2006, Dr. Kahn co-founded the "One Health Initiative," a movement to forge collaborations among physicians, veterinarians, and other scientific-health and environmentally related disciplines. Dr. Kahn actively promotes One Health and engages scientists and the public in pertinent science policy issues in her online column, The Bulletin of the Atomic

Scientists, as well as through numerous journal articles, presentations, and public engagements. She authored the book "Who's in Charge? Leadership during epidemics, bioterror attacks, and other public health crises" and is currently writing a book examining the use of antibiotics in humans and livestock. Dr. Kahn co-organized the Carnegie Corporation's Biodefense Challenge seminar series, which introduces biosecurity, codes of conduct, and dual-use biotech threats to the life sciences community. Dr. Kahn is a fellow of the American College of Physicians and is a recipient of the New Jersey Chapter's Laureate Award.

Dr. Gay Miller, D.V.M., M.S., Ph.D.

Since 1994, Dr. Gay Miller has been a Professor in the Department of Pathobiology at the College of Veterinary Medicine, University of Illinois. She is also a Professor in the Department of Agricultural and Consumer Economics, University of Illinois, and an Adjunct Professor at the Department of Veterinary Population Medicine, University of Minnesota. From 1989 until joining the University of Illinois, Dr. Miller was Associate Professor at the Department of Veterinary Preventive Medicine, Ohio State University. Dr. Miller has more than 30 years of experience in economics and veterinary medicine, bringing a critical economic perspective to problem solving in food safety and disease control. Her primary research focus is on the economic implications of disease outbreaks in food-producing animals, and how different prevention and response strategies can influence both the epidemiological and economic outcomes. In 2006, Dr. Miller was the recipient of an American Association for the Advancement of Science (AAAS) Science and Technology Policy Fellowship, and spent a year working at the United States Department of Agriculture (USDA), providing input into the organization's plans for handling foreign animal diseases, such as avian influenza, that could potentially be introduced into the nation's livestock. Dr. Miller continues to work with the USDA on cooperative agreements. She has authored more than 100 publications and received the Delta Sigma Omicron Distinguished Teaching Award.

Dr. Paul Slovic, Ph.D., M.A.

Dr. Paul Slovic has been a Professor at the Department of Psychology, University of Oregon, since 1986, where he studies judgment and decision processes with an emphasis on decision-making under conditions of risk. In addition, Dr. Slovic is the Founder and President of Decision Research, a nonprofit research organization. As part of his work, Dr. Slovic studies the factors that underlie perceptions of risk and attempts to assess the importance of these perceptions for the management of risk in society. He has developed methods to describe risk perceptions and measure their impacts on individuals, industry, and society. Dr. Slovic has served on the World Economic Forum's Global Agenda Council on Humanitarian Assistance, and the Department of Homeland Security's Steering Committee for the Workshop on Crisis Communication. The author of several hundred publications, his most recent books include "The Perception of Risk," "The Social Amplification of Risk," "The Construction of Preference," and "The Feeling of Risk." Dr. Slovic is a past President of the Society for Risk Analysis, and has received numerous awards including the Society for Risk Analysis Distinguished Achievement Award, the American Psychological Association Distinguished Scientific Contribution Award, the Oregon Academy of Science Outstanding Contribution to Science Award, and the Franklin V. Taylor Lifetime Achievement in Applied Experimental and Engineering Psychology Award.

Dr. Richard Williams, Ph.D., M.A.

Dr. Richard Williams is the Director of Policy Research at the Mercatus Center at George Mason University. Prior to joining the Mercatus Center, he served for 27 years as the Director for Social Sciences at the Center for Food Safety and Applied Nutrition in the U.S. Food and Drug Administration He also served as an adviser to the Harvard Center for Risk Analysis and taught economics at Washington and Lee University. Dr. Williams is a U.S. Army veteran who served in Vietnam. Dr. Williams is an expert in benefit-cost analysis and risk analysis, particularly associated with food safety and nutrition. He has led study teams of multidisciplinary social scientists producing consumer research, risk assessments, and benefit-cost analysis of food safety and nutrition. Additionally, Dr. Williams has created food safety risk analysis classes taught internationally to thousands of public and private scholars and managers, has lectured internationally on risk analysis and economics of nutrition and food safety, and has created federal workgroup-to-peer review of regulatory impact analyses. Dr, Williams has published in journals such as Risk Analysis and the Journal of Policy Analysis and Management and has addressed numerous international governments, including the United Kingdom, South Korea, Yugoslavia, and Australia.

Prof. Jakob Zinsstag, D.V.M., Ph.D., Dip.ECVPH

Since 1998, Prof. Jakob Zinsstag has led a research unit at the Swiss Tropical and Public Health Institute in Basel, investigating the interface of human and animal health, with a focus on the health of nomadic people and control of zoonoses in developing countries under the paradigm of One Health. He is also a Professor of Epidemiology at the University of Basel. From 1990 until his current appointment,

Prof. Zinsstag led a livestock research project at the International Trypanotolerance Centre in The Gambia, and then directed the Centre Suisse de Recherches Scientifiques in Abidjan, Côte d'Ivoire. Prof. Zinsstag's research has been a key factor in validating the One Health concept, and in 2004 he and his team received the TD-award, a Swiss-academies award for transdisciplinary research. His research group is currently part of the Swiss National Centre of Competence in Research North-South, wherein Prof. Zinsstag is Co-leader of Health Research, which has projects based on four continents. Prof. Zinsstag is also Vice President of the International Association for Ecology & Health, Associate Editor of PLoS, Neglected Tropical Diseases, a diplomate of the European College of Veterinary Public Health, and member of the scientific advisory board of the Prince Leopold Institute of Tropical Medicine in Antwerp, Belgium.

Biographical information of ISGP Board of Directors

Dr. George Atkinson, Chairman

Dr. George Atkinson is the founder and Executive Director of the Institute on Science for Global Policy (ISGP) and is an Emeritus Professor of Chemistry, Biochemistry, and Optical Science at the University of Arizona. His professional career has involved academic teaching, research, and administration, roles as a corporate founder and executive, and public service at the federal level. He is former head of the Department of Chemistry at the University of Arizona, the founder of a laser sensor company serving the semiconductor industry, and Science and Technology Adviser (STAS) to U.S. Secretaries of State Colin Powell and Condoleezza Rice. Based on principles derived from his personal experiences, he launched the ISGP in 2008 as a new type of international forum in which credible experts provide governmental and societal leaders with the objective understanding of the science and technology that can be reasonably anticipated to help shape the increasingly global societies of the 21st century. Dr. Atkinson has received National Science Foundation and National Institutes of Health graduate fellowships, a National Academy of Sciences Post Doctoral Fellowship, a Senior Fulbright Award, the SERC Award (U.K.), the Senior Alexander von Humboldt Award (Germany), a Lady Davis Professorship (Israel), the first American Institute of Physics' Scientist Diplomat Award, a Titular Director of the International Union of Pure and Applied Chemistry, the Distinguished Service Award (Indiana University), an Honorary Doctorate (Eckerd College), the Distinguished Achievement Award (University of California, Irvine), and was selected by students as the Outstanding Teacher at the University of Arizona. He received his B.S. (high honors, Phi Beta Kappa) from Eckerd College and his Ph.D. in physical chemistry from Indiana University.

Ms. Loretta Peto, Secretary/Treasurer

Loretta Peto is the Founder and Managing Member at Peto & Company CPA's PLLC. She has experience in: consulting on business valuation and litigation, including valuing businesses for buy-sell agreements, estate and gift tax, marital dissolution and employee compensation; consulting with closely held businesses regarding business restructure, cash management, succession planning, performance enhancement and business growth; and managing tax-related projects, including specialty areas in corporate, partnership, estate and gift tax, business reorganizations, and multistate tax reporting. She is a Certified Public Accountant and accredited in Business Valuations. She is a member of the Finance Committee and Chair of the Audit Committee at Tucson Regional Economic Opportunities. She also is a member of the DM50 and Tucson Pima Arts Council. She received a Master of Accounting - Emphasis in Taxation degree from the University of Arizona in 1984, and was awarded the Outstanding Graduate Student Award.

Dr. Janet Bingham, Member

Dr. Janet Bingham has been President and CEO and a consultant to the Huntsman Cancer Foundation (HCF) since 2006. The foundation is a charitable organization that provides financial support to the Huntsman Cancer Institute, the largest cancer specialty research center and hospital in the Intermountain West. Dr. Bingham also has managed Huntsman Cancer Biotechnology Inc. In addition, she was appointed Executive Vice President and Chief Operating Officer with the Huntsman Foundation in 2008. The Huntsman Foundation is the private charitable foundation established by Jon M. Huntsman Sr. to support education, cancer interests, programs for abused women and children, and programs for the homeless. Before joining the Huntsman philanthropic organizations, Dr. Bingham was the Vice President for External Relations and Advancement at The University of Arizona. Prior to her seven years as a UA vice president, she served as Assistant Vice President for Health Sciences at The University of Arizona Health Sciences Center. Dr. Bingham was recognized as one of the Ten Most Powerful Women in Arizona.

Dr. Henry Koffler, Member

Dr. Henry Koffler is President Emeritus of the University of Arizona (UA). He served as President of the UA from 1982-1991. From 1982 he also held professorships in the Departments of Biochemistry, Molecular and Cellular Biology, and Microbiology and Immunology, positions from which he retired in 1997 as Professor Emeritus of Biochemistry. His personal research during these years concentrated on the physiology and molecular biology of microorganisms. He was Vice President for Academic Affairs, University of Minnesota, and Chancellor, University of Massachusetts/Amherst, before coming to the UA. He taught at Purdue University, where he was a Hovde Distinguished Professor, and the School of Medicine at Western Reserve University (now Case Western Reserve University). Dr. Koffler served as a founding governor and founding vice-chairman of the American Academy of Microbiology, and as a member of the governing boards of Fermi National Accelerator Laboratory, the Argonne National Laboratory, and the Superconducting Super Collider Laboratory. He was also a board member of the Association of American Colleges and Universities, a member and chairman of the Council of Presidents and a member of the executive committee of the National

Association of Land Grant Colleges and Universities. He was also Founder, President and board member of The Arizona Senior Academy, the driving force in the development of the Academy Village, an innovative living and learning community. Among the honors that Dr. Koffler has received are a Guggenheim Fellowship and the Eli Lilly Award in Bacteriology and Immunology.

Dr. Charles Parmenter, Member
Dr. Charles Parmenter is a Distinguished Professor Emeritus of Chemistry at Indiana University. He also served as Professor and Assistant and Associate Professor at Indiana University in a career there that spanned nearly half a century (1964-2010). He earned his bachelor's degree from the University of Pennsylvania and served as a Lieutenant in the U.S. Air Force from 1955-57. He worked at DuPont after serving the military and received his Ph.D. from the University of Rochester and was a Postdoctoral Fellow at Harvard University. He has been elected a Member of the National Academy of Sciences and the American Academy of Arts and Sciences; and a Fellow of the American Physical Society and the American Association for the Advancement of Science. He was a Guggenheim Fellow, a Fulbright Senior Scholar, and received the Senior Alexander von Humboldt Award in 1984. He has received the Earle K Plyler Prize, was a Spiers Medalist and Lecturer at the Faraday Society, and served as Chair of the Division of Physical Chemistry of the American Chemical Society, Co-Chair of the First Gordon Conference on Molecular Energy Transfer, Co-organizer of the Telluride Workshop on Large Amplitude Motion and Molecular Dynamics, and Councilor of Division of Chemical Physics, American Physical Society.

Biographical information of ISGP staff

Dr. George Atkinson, Executive Director

Dr. George Atkinson is the founder and Executive Director of the Institute on Science for Global Policy (ISGP) and is an Emeritus Professor of Chemistry, Biochemistry, and Optical Science at the University of Arizona. His professional career has involved academic teaching, research, and administration, roles as a corporate founder and executive, and public service at the federal level. He is former head of the Department of Chemistry at the University of Arizona, the founder of a laser sensor company serving the semiconductor industry, and Science and Technology Adviser (STAS) to U.S. Secretaries of State Colin Powell and Condoleezza Rice. Based on principles derived from his personal experiences, he launched the ISGP in 2008 as a new type of international forum in which credible experts provide governmental and societal leaders with the objective understanding of the science and technology that can be reasonably anticipated to help shape the increasingly global societies of the 21st century. Dr. Atkinson has received National Science Foundation and National Institutes of Health graduate fellowships, National Academy of Sciences Post Doctoral Fellowship, Senior Fulbright Award, the SERC Award (U.K.), the Senior Alexander von Humboldt Award (Germany), a Lady Davis Professorship (Israel), the first American Institute of Physics' Scientist Diplomat Award, a Titular Director of the International Union of Pure and Applied Chemistry, the Distinguished Service Award (Indiana University), an Honorary Doctorate (Eckerd College), the Distinguished Achievement Award (University of California, Irvine), and was selected by students as the Outstanding Teacher at the University of Arizona. He received his B.S. (high honors, Phi Beta Kappa) from Eckerd College and his Ph.D. in physical chemistry from Indiana University.

Jennifer Boice, M.B.A.

Jennifer Boice is the Program Manager of the ISGP. Prior to this role, Ms. Boice worked for 25 years in the newspaper industry, primarily at the Tucson Citizen and briefly at USA Today. She was the Editor of the Tucson Citizen when it was closed in 2009. Additional appointments at the Tucson Citizen included Business News Editor, Online Department head and Senior Editor. She also was a columnist. Ms. Boice received an M.B.A. from the University of Arizona and graduated from Pomona College in California with a degree in economics.

Alexis Boyd, M.Sc.
Alexis Boyd is a Senior Fellow with the ISGP. In addition, she is currently pursuing her Ph.D. in the Institute of Biomedical Sciences, Department of Microbiology and Immunology at The George Washington University. Her research is focused on the immune response to helminth parasites. Previously, Ms. Boyd was an Infectious Disease Training Fellow at the Centers for Disease Control and Prevention in the Division of Parasitology. She received her M.Sc. in Public Health Microbiology from the The George Washington University and majored in biotechnology at Rutgers University.

Melanie Brickman Stynes, Ph.D., M.Sc.
Melanie Brickman Stynes is Associate Director with the ISGP. As a researcher focused on the juncture of public health, demography, policy, and geography, she bridges multiple fields in her emerging and persistent infectious diseases research. Her work has paid particular attention to issues surrounding tuberculosis control (historic and contemporary). She is also an Adjunct Professor at Baruch College's School of Public Affairs in New York City. Additionally, Dr. Brickman Stynes spent nearly a decade as a Research Associate for the Center for International Earth Science Information Network (CIESIN) of Columbia University, where she worked on a range of projects related to health, disease, poverty, urbanization, and population issues. She received her Ph.D. in medical geography from University College London and her M.Sc. in medical demography from the London School of Hygiene and Tropical Medicine.

Sweta Chakraborty, Ph.D.
Sweta Chakraborty is a Senior Fellow with the ISGP. She recently completed post-doctoral research on pharmaceutical regulation and product liability at Oxford University's Centre for Socio-Legal Studies and remains an active member of Wolfson College. Dr. Chakraborty received her doctorate in Risk Management from King's College London and has helped to design and co-teach a summer course in London on Managing Hazards in Europe and the United States with Indiana University's School of Public and Environmental Affairs. Her undergraduate degrees are in Decision Science and International Relations from Carnegie Mellon University.

Jill Fromewick, Sc.D., M.S.
Jill Fromewick is Senior Scientific Consultant with the ISGP. A social epidemiologist by training, Dr. Fromewick maintains a dual focus on quantitative and qualitative methods. Her research spans a broad range of public health topics, primarily

focused on investigating the impact of state and local policy on health and health disparities. She is the founder and Executive Director of Sparrow Research Group, a global public health consulting firm specializing in program design, evaluation, and social science research. Dr. Fromewick holds Master's and Doctor of Science degrees from the Department of Society, Human Development, and Health at the Harvard School of Public Health.

Jung Joo "JJ" Hwang, Ph.D., M.S., Pharm.D.

JJ Hwang is Consultant, Synthetic Biology, with the ISGP. Dr. Hwang is a Consultant to the BioAtla, LLC and currently enrolled in a master's program at the University of California San Diego International Relations/Pacific Study, specializing in international public policy with a focus on global health. She has been a Scientific Director and Lab Head at Samsung Advanced Institute of Technology, a Scientific Director at Protedyne Inc., a Senior Scientist at MitoKor, and an Assistant Professor of Biochemistry and Molecular Biology at the University of Southern California, while managing various projects on biomarker/drug/diagnostic chip development. She received her Ph.D. in Biochemistry at the University of Pittsburgh School of Medicine and her M.S. and Pharm.D. from the Ewha Womans University in South Korea.

Anna Isaacs, M.Sc.

Anna Isaacs is a Senior Fellow with the ISGP. She has previously focused on minority health issues and is experienced in field- and desk-based qualitative research. She has interned as a researcher at a variety of nonprofit institutions and also at the House of Commons in London. Ms. Isaacs received her M.Sc. with distinction in Medical Anthropology from University College London and a B.Sc. in Political Science from the University of Bristol.

David Miller, M.B.A.

David Miller is a Scientific/Program Consultant with the ISGP. Previously, he was Director, Medical Advocacy, Policy and Patient Programs at GlaxoSmithKline, where he led the company's U.S. efforts relating to science policy. In this role, he advised senior management on policy issues, and was the primary liaison between the company and the national trade associations, Pharmaceutical Research and Manufacturers of America (PhRMA) and Biotechnology Industry Organization (BIO). He also held management positions in business development and quality assurance operations. Mr. Miller received his B.S. in Chemistry and his M.B.A. from the University of North Carolina at Chapel Hill.

Sarah Rhodes, Ph.D.

Sarah Rhodes is a Fellow with ISGP, and a Research Fellow at the National Institutes of Health (NIH), where her duties are split between active research and a policy analyst position at the Office of Autism Research Coordination. A neuroscientist by training, Dr. Rhodes' research focuses on teasing apart the involvement of different brain regions in goal-directed behavior, which is disrupted in a range of neuropsychological disorders. Prior to moving to the United States and joining NIH, Dr. Rhodes was a postdoctoral Research Associate at Cardiff University, United Kingdom, where she coordinated a joint grant with University College London. Dr. Rhodes holds a M.A. in (Biological) Natural Sciences from Cambridge University, and a Ph.D. in Behavioral Neuroscience from Cardiff University.

Arthur Rotstein, M.S.J.

Arthur Rotstein is an editor with the ISGP. Prior to joining the ISGP, Mr. Rotstein worked for the Washington D.C. Daily News, held a fellowship at the University of Chicago, and spent more than 35 years working as a journalist with The Associated Press. His writings have covered diverse topics that include politics, immigration, border issues, heart transplant and artificial heart developments, Biosphere 2, college athletics, features, papal visits, and the Mexico City earthquake. Mr. Rotstein holds a bachelor's degree in journalism from the University of Missouri and a M.S.J. from Northwestern University's Medill School of Journalism.

Raymond Schmidt, Ph.D.

Ray Schmidt is a Senior Fellow with the ISGP. In addition, he is a physical chemist/chemical engineer with a strong interest in organizational effectiveness and community health care outcomes. While teaching at the university level, his research focused on using laser light scattering to study liquids, polymer flow, and biological transport phenomena. Upon moving to the upstream petroleum industry, he concentrated on research and development (R&D) and leading multidisciplinary teams from numerous companies to investigate future enhanced oil recovery ideas and to pilot/commercialize innovative recovery methods in domestic and foreign locations. Dr. Schmidt received his Ph.D. in chemistry from Emory University.

Ramiro Soto

Ramiro Soto is an office assistant at the ISGP. He currently is an undergraduate student at the University of Arizona College of Science seeking a Bachelor of Science degree in General Applied Mathematics. Beyond his academic curriculum, Mr. Soto is an active member of the Pride of Arizona marching band since 2010 and recently became a member of the athletic pep band. He completed an internship with the Walt Disney Company Parks and Resorts segment in 2011. After completing his undergraduate education, he plans to apply for a doctoral program furthering his studies in Mathematics.

Matt Wenham, D.Phil.

Matt Wenham is Associate Director with the ISGP. He formerly was a postdoctoral research fellow at the National Institutes of Health in Bethesda, Maryland. His research involved studying the interaction of protein toxins produced by pathogenic E. coli strains with human cells. Dr. Wenham received his D. Phil. from the Sir William Dunn School of Pathology, University of Oxford, United Kingdom, where he was a Rhodes Scholar. Prior to this, he worked in research positions at universities in Adelaide and Melbourne, Australia. Dr. Wenham received his bachelor's and honours degrees in biochemistry from the University of Adelaide, South Australia, and holds a Graduate Diploma of Education from Monash University, Victoria.